MANPOWER PLANNING IN THE NATIONAL HEALTH SERVICE

Manpower Planning in the National Health Service

Edited by

A. F. LONG

*Nuffield Centre for Health Service Studies,
University of Leeds*

and

G. MERCER

*Department of Sociology,
University of Leeds*

Gower

Published by
Gower Publishing Company Limited,
Westmead, Farnborough, Hampshire, England

ISBN O 566 00425 9

Printed in Great Britain by Biddles Ltd, Guildford, Surrey

Contents

List of Contributors

M. Blunt   Assistant Secretary (Manpower Planning),
Trent RHA

J. Cree   STAMP Training Officer,
Wessex RHA

P. Dixon   Regional Manpower Planning Officer,
Wessex RHA

S. Harrison   Lecturer,
Nuffield Centre for Health Services Studies,
The University of Leeds

A. F. Long*   Lecturer,
Nuffield Centre for Health Services Studies,
The University of Leeds

E. McAleavey   Senior Manpower Planning Officer,
West Midlands RHA

G. Mercer*   Lecturer,
Department of Sociology,
The University of Leeds

S. Naylor   Operational Research Officer,
West Midlands RHA

R. Petch   Assistant Secretary, DHSS
formerly Head of Manpower Intelligence Branch,
DHSS

*Joint Editors of this Volume

Acknowledgements

As joint editors of this volume we are pleased to acknowledge the advice and assistance that has supported its compilation and completion. The World Health Organisation granted us permission to use material from: T.L.Hall and A.Mejia (eds), *Health Manpower Planning: Principles, Methods, Issues*, World Health Organisation, Geneva 1978. The University of Leeds provided a research grant that enabled us to conduct a field study of manpower planning and interview health service officials around the country. The co-operation of those with whom we have been in contact has been generous and helpful throughout. The general form and content of the book has benefited from the constructive criticism of Robin Gourlay. Last, but not least, the excellent typing and organisational skills of Jane Thompson have seen the project completed on time.

Andrew Long and Geoffrey Mercer
The University of Leeds, 1980

1 Context and Priorities

A. F. Long and G. Mercer

The objective of this book is to explore current manpower planning
practice in the National Health Service in England. This topic has
assumed a growing significance in health sector policy making, and much
heralded steps have been taken in recent years to design a planning
system that will formalise a role for manpower planning. With the NHS
again under close review, manpower questions have been subject to more
rigorous scrutiny. Thus the Royal Commission on the NHS was set up in
1976 with a remit, 'to consider in the interests of both patients and
those who work in the National Health Service the best use and management of the financial and *manpower* resources of the NHS'. (1) (emphasis
added)

That a major rethink of the NHS should be deemed necessary so soon
after the 1974 reorganisation bears witness to the number of critics
and the level of disenchantment with the present system of health care.
'Whichever way you look at it the NHS over the past five years has
never had it so bad,' (2) summarises an all too popular viewpoint.
Harsh and often much exaggerated though such pronouncements are, the
NHS has never been short of detractors. Indeed, statements about
current deficiencies closely resemble the criticism directed against
the pre-NHS system. Then there were complaints about the shortages in
facilities and trained staff, the unsatisfactory conditions for patient
treatment and care, the inefficient organisation of the services, their
inequitable distribution round the country, and the lack of funds for
expansion. (3) Together with these perennial grievances, the
problems of industrial relations, private medicine, and wider
participation in the running of the service illustrate the spread of
contemporary issues. This 'condition of the NHS' debate constitutes a
wide ranging and well rehearsed discussion about what the NHS should be
doing, and how it might be administered more effectively and
efficiently.

Although always faced by insufficient finance and resources
generally, the NHS had become accustomed to continued growth in health
care spending, and according to Regional Administrators, 'the result
has been to allow slack management, with no incentive to examine
obsolete patterns of spending, or to develop a coherent plan for the
future'. (4) Current economic difficulties have encouraged fresh

1

policies, and a strong momentum has been established to inject more cost consciousness into health service management. Since three quarters of health expenditure goes on manpower, it is no surprise that manpower planning has been spawned as one of the more ambitious offspring of this pressure.

Most commentators on the progress of manpower planning in the NHS to date have been less than enthusiastic. The Royal Commission ventured a gentle rebuff, 'that a more positive approach to manpower planning generally is required', but this has been translated by others to mean that current practice is 'appalling'. (5) This book examines the state of NHS manpower planning against that backcloth of criticism and disappointment. What is being attempted, why, by whom, and with what consequences? To set the discussion in perspective, this chapter outlines the development and formative influences on manpower planning in the NHS.

COSTS AND MANPOWER IN THE NHS

There has been a massive growth in state expenditure in Britain since the first World War; it rose from 12.7 per cent of gross national product (GNP) in 1910, through 44.9 per cent in 1951, to 57.9 per cent in 1975. Within this total, the proportion devoted to health services has risen marginally to the 5.7 per cent level in 1975, although the pace of spending has quickened with health costs quadrupling between 1949 and 1969, and again in the ten years since then. (6) Nevertheless as much as three quarters of this extra finance has been swallowed up in rising costs. As a labour intensive service the NHS has been hard hit by wage inflation. At the same time the demand for health care has not abated; instead with the significant ageing of the country's population it has increased. (7)

International comparisons reveal that the UK allocates a smaller proportion of its gross domestic product (GDP) to health services than any other advanced industrial society - with the exception of Japan. However there is a lack of a clear relationship between financial input and health output on the one hand, or between input and medical or nursing manpower on the other hand. For example, West Germany spends 6.7 per cent of its GDP on health services which places it in the middle of the international league. Yet it combines a high doctor-population ratio with a low nurse-population ratio, low life expectancy, high perinatal and maternal mortality. Although the figures within the UK vary, in England and Wales despite the relatively low financial input compared with West Germany, and the much lower ratio of doctors, life expectancy, perinatal and maternal mortality figures are all much better. (8)

In absolute terms the NHS budget amounted to nearly £7,000 million in 1977, and in the parlous condition of the British economy it has not been difficult to depict this mushrooming health bill as an unacceptable burden. Britain has experienced an increase in inflation, in unemployment and trade deficits, while at the same time GNP, industrial production and the share of world trade have all failed to improve or compensate for difficulties elsewhere in the economy. In a search for causes, orthodox Keynesian economics has been under attack, and blame attached to 'excessive' and 'unproductive' state expenditure. In consequence, the NHS is expected to hold, if not cut its spending. (9)

Notwithstanding the widespread public support which the health service enjoys, there are major difficulties in reducing health expenditure.   Contrary to the expectations of many involved with the establishment of the NHS the demand for health care has not diminished after the initial years of adjustment to a service free at the point of delivery.   Instead the prevailing opinion accepts that 'demand will always be one jump ahead' of the supply of health services.   In the pursuit of a comprehensive and more effective service, costs have spiralled as methods of treatment have grown increasingly complex and expensive.   Merely to maintain current standards entails a one per cent annual increase in real terms.   The NHS is in the unenviable position of having to spend more just to stand still. (10)

The NHS is further hindered because as a labour intensive, personal service industry, its unit costs have grown relatively faster than in other sectors.   The budget is dominated by the wages and salaries bill. This jumped from 58.9 per cent of total costs in 1954-55, to nearly 75 per cent in 1976-77. (11)   In 1977, the numbers employed by the health service topped the one million mark, as a whole time equivalent, and in England alone the figure totalled 800,000.   DHSS projections for the period 1976-86 envisaged that the percentage of the employed population in the NHS in England will increase from 3.6 to 4 per cent, assuming a 1.5 per cent annual revenue growth rate.   The composition of the workforce in England and Wales includes significant numbers of highly trained personnel: in 1977 43 per cent of staff were nurses, 9 per cent doctors and dentists, and slightly over 6 per cent in the professional and technical groups.   Overall, the NHS has a predominantly female workforce, although there is an uneven distribution across staff groups - from 88 per cent of nurses, and 66 per cent of ancillary staff to only 18 per cent of medical and dental practitioners. The NHS also relies heavily on part time staff, who constitute about one third of all employees, although these are concentrated in the ancillary and nursing populations. (12)

The number of NHS staff has more than doubled in the period since 1949, although unevenly across and within groups.   These trends are illustrated for the period 1949 to 1974 in Table 1.1, and since reorganisation in Table 1.2.   Over the 30 years since 1949, professional and technical staff have trebled in number, doctors and nurses doubled, while ancillary grades have grown least - by 50 per cent.   In some cases, as with doctors and dentists, the increase has been most evident among hospital staff where the career structure has opened up ·to provide a higher percentage of senior (consultant) posts. Against this, the trend elsewhere has often been towards the greater use of aides and unqualified staff.   Thus within the nursing category the proportion of untrained staff has swelled from 20 to 30 per cent. (13) Overall, the growth in NHS employees quickened in the 1970s, with the exception again of the ancillary grades.

The NHS has not made headway in reducing its manpower; neither has much been attempted in the area of redeployment.   Attempts to bolster managerial control through the adoption of well tried techniques of work study from private industry have only made an impact on the

Table 1.1

Staffing in the NHS: England and Wales, Whole-Time Equivalents[a]

Staff Group	1949	1959	1969	1974[b]	1974	1977
i) Hospital Medical	11,735	16,033	22,001	26,527	26,527	29,517
ii) General Medical Practitioners[c]	18,000	22,091	21,505	22,885	22,885	23,721
iii) Hospital Dental	206	444	723	824	824	932
iv) General Dental Practitioners[c]	9,425	10,418	10,659	11,528	11,528	12,360
v) Nurses and Midwives	135,000	181,000	245,889	289,953	324,783	362,618
vi) Professional and Technical	12,840	20,171	30,669	39,763	46,288	57,367
vii) Ancillary	120,000	150,000	170,880	169,792	173,847	184,198
viii) Administrative and Clerical	23,797	30,270	43,328	59,668	88,011	104,939
ix) All Staff	331,003	430,427	545,654	620,847	694,693	775,643

Notes

[a] Figures are given to the nearest unit. All figures relate to 30 September of the year in question.

[b] Until 1974 figures for staff in lines v) to ix) relate to hospital staff. Thereafter they are only available in terms of all employees in the Health Service.

[c] Numbers not whole-time equivalents.

Source
DHSS, Staffing of the National Health Service (England), March 1979, Table 4.

4

Table 1.2

Indices of Staff Growth: England and Wales

Staff Group	1949 = 100[a]			1974 = 100[b]	
	1959	1969	1974	1977	
Hospital Medical	137	187	226	111	
General Medical Practitioners	123	119	127	104	
Hospital Dental	216	351	400	113	
General Dental Practitioners	111	113	122	107	
Nurses and Midwives	134	182	215	112	
Professional and Technical	157	239	310	124	
Ancillary	125	142	141	106	
Administrative and Clerical	127	178	251	119	
All Staff	130	165	188	112	

Notes

[a] All figures relate to hospital staff only.

[b] All figures relate to all employees in the Health Service.

Source

As for Table 1.1.

ancillary grades, where the reduction in numbers has been associated with the introduction of bonus schemes. In addition, and perhaps not unconnected, trade union membership and industrial disputes have risen particularly in this group of staff. (14) In general, the substitution of capital for labour, and the more flexible deployment of labour itself, are instruments to achieve a more optimum balance of resources. But initiatives of this sort are confronted by several obstacles. A primary difficulty rests in the determination of the efficiency of different forms of treatment or in assessing the productivity of personal services workers. (15) Policies in this area threaten the more recently unionised employees, as well as the autonomy of more established professional groups. Redeployment of the labour force has foundered on growing sectional rivalries between staff groups, the increasing fragmentation of occupational categories, and the more ready resort to industrial action to protect staff interests.

> 'It is easier to advocate flexibility than to achieve it. The
> heavy investment in existing personnel, training syllabuses and
> institutions, Whitley Council agreements and professional codes
> of practice ensures that even the most marginal changes in
> activity are often extremely difficult to achieve. Staff may
> feel that their jobs are at risk, particularly in times of high
> unemployment, and that their status may be eroded if their
> functions are not jealously guarded. In a few cases there may
> be legal problems.' (16)

However, the health service budget has profited from the generally low rates of pay offered in comparison with equivalent staff in private industry, or abroad. (17) Steps to overcome this inheritance have been taken with the implementation of the recommendations of the Pay Comparability Commission proposals, and the NHS manpower bill must inevitably mount. (18) In sum, there are major barriers to managerial action to control the expansion in expenditure, and the climate is less than conducive to positive manpower planning, although without it costs cannot be significantly controlled.

ADMINISTRATIVE REFORM

If the features outlined above have not made for an easy growth of manpower planning in the NHS, administrative reorganisation in 1974 created fresh possibilities. Popular conceptions of the origins and objectives of the NHS emphasise the intention to create a service geared to public need rather than individual ability to pay. It is often ignored that a crucial objective in the 1940s was the development of a more rational planning and organisation of health care which led to a quasi-nationalisation of the health services. That same thinking underlay the reorganisation of the NHS in 1974. (19)

The DHSS identified the following principles as central to the overhaul of the management of the NHS:

> 'the integral involvement of the health care professions in
> planning and management at all levels of the service;
>
> decentralisation and delegation of decision making but

within policies established at a higher level;

a territorial structure and organisational mechanisms which allowed closer collaboration with local authorities and facilitated joint planning and working on matters of common concern;

provision for effective central control over the money spent in the service to enable the Secretary of State to discharge responsibilities laid upon him by Parliament.' (20)

This constituted a second stage in the 'nationalisation' of the health service, since a formal structure was designed to unify the several parts, and the various levels at which care was provided. A single service also opened the way for comprehensive and co-ordinated manpower planning policies.

The need for reform has been advanced in a stream of official reports. The main impetus crystallised around the rising philosophy of corporate management and planning, which advocates enhanced rationality in corporate operations and structures. It was an attempt to inject ideas and methods from private industry into the public sector. Not that health was the only domain of public administration engulfed by an enthusiasm for corporate planning. Important landmarks included: the 1966 Salmon Report on the administration of nursing; the Seebohm Report in 1968 on the social services; and successive reports on local government which culminated in the Local Government Act of 1972. (21) The latter outlined major alterations in boundaries and structures which gave greater immediacy to the impending NHS reorganisation. At the base of this scheme was a three-fold tier system - DHSS, Regional and Area Health Authorities (RHAs and AHAs), and supplemented by health districts which constituted the operational context for health care. These reforms were complemented by a new organisational climate for policy making as laid down by the corporate planning system. The official rhetoric claimed to balance the centripetal forces contained in the notion of local control, following delegation from the DHSS, with a centralised co-ordination of activities across the tiers. To many observers this presaged a tight rather than a loose structure.

Notwithstanding disagreement about the locus of power, the launching of the reorganised service stimulated management to designate manpower problems a high place in the planning pecking order, along with finance and capital. While the DHSS sought to maintain its considerable economic clout, there has been some latitude for manoeuvre in health authority policy making which has hindered central orchestration of the manpower front. 'Because of the size and complexity of the NHS budget, it would not be practicable for DHSS to control expenditure in great detail.' (22) The maldistribution of resources across the country has however resulted in initiatives from the centre which have a consequential impact on manpower resources through the Regions. In England the Resource Allocation Working Party (RAWP) recommended in 1976 a different basis for allocating revenue and capital funds. Previous methods were criticised because of the favourable treatment of metropolitan Regions - essentially for historical reasons rather than current health needs. (23) Whatever the imperfections of the RAWP formula, its potential influence on the distribution of NHS manpower is self-evident.

The DHSS has also tried to lead the service by detailing long term
aims in health care. The publication of *Priorities for Health and
Personal Social Services* was regarded as a new departure for the DHSS,
although it broadly codified the views contained in previous White
Papers. (24) It spelt out, in general terms, the main areas of growth
as services for the elderly, the mentally ill and handicapped, and
children. Primary health care in the community was a particular target
for improvement. Once again the influx of resources to these care
groups had clear manpower implications. Apart from services to
children, all of those listed had experienced difficulty in recruiting
staff and had relied heavily on immigrant labour. Again, community
services have been unevenly developed and could not cope with much
increased service responsibilities. (25) This constituted a severe
test for the NHS planning system, as it was charged with shifting
resources to the priority areas against a background of financial
restrictions.

The question arises whether, and in what ways, the quality of NHS
manpower planning has been affected by these trends. Have the
administrative reforms of recent years created a radical managerial
rethink across the service in terms of forward planning, priority
definition and resource allocation? Manpower was in theory high on the
agenda of health service planning. It remained to be seen whether the
practice in the service had been similarly reformed and revitalised.

THE EXPERIENCE OF MANPOWER PLANNING

Economic pressures and administrative reforms combined to elevate
manpower planning from relative obscurity to a position of formal
significance. If the 1970s now seem a watershed, recognition is due to
the albeit often tentative and piecemeal steps taken since the inception
of the NHS. Manpower planning to obtain the appropriate mix of staff
in the right place when it was wanted had attracted the attention of NHS
managers in earlier years. Previous excursions into this field should
not be lambasted as outright failures. (26) This is not to excuse
their lack of foresight. It has to be recognised that the problems
confronting the NHS are complex and not easily overcome. Manpower has
long been accepted as a costly ingredient that needed to be controlled,
and misalignments in the supply and demand for staff have been
deprecated. There was not the apparent sensitivity to these problems
that now characterises the service. (27) The usual reaction, as the
NHS lurched periodically, was a Royal Commission or an official working
party. Shegog has aptly summed up these typically British responses,
'to the need for thinking aloud about government policy. But such
bodies possess only discontinuous, sometimes amateur, powers of analysis
and their method precludes long-term investigation.' (28)

Most frequent attention has been accorded to medical manpower, since
this group has always been regarded as the lynchpin of any health
service. (29) More intermittent concern has been given to nursing
staff, particularly towards the trained grades, although since the
Briggs Report of 1972, interest has been directed to the possibility of
increasing the contribution and number of nursing aides. (30) Other

occupational groups have been much neglected. It was not until the
1960s that a series of inquiries extended the perspective - for example,
to scientific staff, engineers, administrators and paramedical staff.
(31) Not that all of the reports have come directly under the aegis of
the DHSS. Most notably, the National Board for Prices and Incomes
issued wide ranging reviews of nursing and ancillary staff. (32)

The level of sophistication of these studies varied considerably.
Not always fairly, the enduring impression has been the inaccuracy of
their forecasts. (33) The usual recommendations encompassed calls for
an improvement in staff education and training, and demands that a
career in the health service be made more attractive to entice good
quality recruits. This entailed higher remuneration, better working
conditions and a more open career structure at the higher levels.
These measures were deemed the most likely to enhance recruitment and
retention of staff, although the NHS has not met with particular success
in this area.

As demonstrated in innumerable critiques of medical manpower reports,
the analysis has been restricted to the stock of British doctors, and
has ignored or played down the impact of flows between grades, across
countries, or mobility in and out of work - as with those who are
looking after a family. (34) Reviews of medical manpower were also
distinctive because of their concern with the overproduction of
personnel, whereas most other groups - at least until recently - have
started from the premise that they had to concentrate their efforts into
stimulating recruitment. Again, while most planning for medics was
conducted on a national plane, the DHSS took a far less significant role
in planning overall levels, or the distribution of other staff groups.

The Royal Commission summarised the haphazard estimation of demand for
labour as follows:

'It is impossible with our present state of knowledge to say how
many workers the NHS needs and of what type: roles are not
always clearly defined, the level of training required may not
be clear, and the difficulty of establishing standards of
quality . . . is reflected in the absence of generally accepted
staffing standards.

This lack also makes it difficult to monitor effectively over-
and under-manning even locally. Nor do international
comparisons of staffing offer much guidance. Finally,
calculations about the numbers of staff needed must take
account of their relative cost and the availability of cash
to pay them. The aim should be to provide as much good
quality care as possible from a given budget.' (35)

In consequence, estimates of demand for manpower have found little
common ground, beyond the time-honoured assumption that the present
level of staffing was inadequate and should be improved. In most
circumstances the need was derived from official professional opinion
although severely constrained by economic conditions.

In more recent reports the quality of forecasting has been bolstered,
in appearance if not in reality, by increasingly complex model building

exercises. As yet the techniques associated with operational research have made slow progress in health manpower planning, and the MANPLAN suite of complex computerised routines has been greatly underused - both for the want of interested planners and suitable data, and not a little suspicion in the NHS of the practical benefit to be gained at the operational level. (36) To date, the most available illustrations of these techniques are contained in the Scottish Home and Health Department (SHHD) reports on nurses, and parallel work on administrative staff south of the border contained in the Hoare Report. (37)

Whatever the path followed or recommended by these excursions into manpower planning, pressure grew on the DHSS to adopt a more active role. The Merrison Report reinforced these views, and appealed for a more interventionist stance to ensure that priority programmes among nursing and medical staff were instituted. (38)

It should not be forgotten however that the qualitative focus on patients' health needs does not always merge easily with the quantitative cost-benefit accounting and operational research techniques that have been advocated in manpower planning. Health care and treatment often defies easy quantification, or at least agreement on the criteria on which the necessary measurement is based.

Furthermore, the DHSS although charged with the overall responsibility for the health service, has often been in a position of something less than complete charge of its own domain. Surveys of the reorganised NHS have reported, 'a great deal of anger and frustration at what many regard as a seriously over-elaborate system of government, administration and decision making. The multiplicity of levels, the over-elaboration of consultative machinery, the inability to get decision making completed nearer the point of delivery of services, and what some describe as unacceptably wasteful use of manpower resources were recurrent themes . . .' (39) Yet many of these current problems pre-date, and will no doubt outlast, future administrative reforms. The following list is by no means exhaustive: '. . . the grave economic difficulties which the country has faced since 1974; the consequent effect on remuneration and the development of the NHS generally; changes in the organisation of nursing following the Salmon Committee Report; the increased unionisation of staff and the development of more "industrial" attitudes; the shortage of personnel officers in the NHS, and the emergence of new professional groups, for example in the laboratories.' (40)

As a part of the public sector, the NHS has been expected to operate as a front line protagonist in recurring battles fought on behalf of governmental policies for wage restraint. Again, in crucial contexts, the DHSS has had nothing more forceful to rely on than its ability to influence and persuade those at the local level. But unlike several nationalised industries the NHS was slow to establish a central personnel function, and there remains much fragmentation across authorities in the responsibility for staff recruitment, training and career development. (41)

From this brief review, health service planning can be seen to have spluttered forward in fits and starts. It has had to endure the combined deficiencies of little recognition, poor information, little

expertise, and innumerable economic, political and social constraints.
Improvement of the administration of its manpower resources has become a
widely promulgated objective of the reformed NHS.   Manpower planning
has acquired both an institutional base - organisationally within the
DHSS and the NHS authorities - and a key function within the new
planning system.   As other chapters in this volume discuss, the
institution within the DHSS of the Manpower Intelligence Branch (MIB),
along with the Joint Manpower Planning and Information Working Group
(MAPLIN), and the prospect of a Standard Manpower Planning and Personnel
Information System (STAMP) - or some similar development - have raised
expectations that manpower planning will secure a wider credibility by
offering an effective contribution to health service policy making.

PLAN OF THE BOOK

Several issues immediately emerge as worthy of detailed elaboration.
There is a range of technical questions about what manpower planning
should entail, and what in practice has been the brief accepted within
the NHS.   Much of the confusion, or difference in interpretation,
arises because of the specific organisational context in which health
service planning is conducted.   It is not always apparent, for example,
who is supposed to be doing what in the various administrative levels.
Even when formal lines of authority have been demarcated, there is dis-
agreement whether the 'natural' place for making manpower policies has
been identified.   The Royal Commission espoused the widely favoured
view that, 'large organisations are most efficient when problems are
solved and decisions taken at the lowest effective point.' (42)
Unfortunately, apart from arguing against a central planning body - with
the exception of doctors and dentists - the Commission neglected to
explore what the several levels of the service might properly regard as
their own province in manpower matters.   Who does what, when and how
constitutes an underlying theme through all of the contributions to this
book.

The approach adopted within the national health service context to
manpower planning needs to be situated against concepts and practices
which have currency in manpower planning generally, although there is no
universally agreed standard by which to rank all initiatives in this
field.   Chapter Two outlines some of the main concepts and issues in
manpower planning, and explores these within the specific organisational
climate of the health service.   In Chapter Three case studies of
manpower planning for the medical, nursing and paramedical professions
are discussed.   Across these three case studies concern centres on the
approach adopted, the methodology developed, the implementation of
proposals, and the lessons learned.   The connecting thread consists of
a requirement on management to explore and include the manpower aspects
of proposals within overall health service decision making and planning.

One of the most frequently stated prerequisites to manpower planning
in the NHS is the need for a comprehensive and easily accessed manpower
data base.   Chapter Four outlines the development of the STAMP system
at Wessex RHA and available to the NHS in July 1980.   Discussion also
examines how manpower information can be utilised for operational
management and planning, to extend the consideration given by managers
and senior officers to the manpower implication of proposals.   Manpower

planning can never be an entirely technical task, and Chapter Five seeks to provide a counterbalance by highlighting some of the economic and political pressures that constrain this activity in the health service.

The focus then turns to the way in which the manpower component has been incorporated within strategic planning and the role performed by the DHSS and the various levels of the NHS. The basic issue of the centralisation or devolution of health manpower underlies the discussion in the next three chapters. The place of the centre in developing manpower planning in the NHS is identified in Chapter Six. Chapter Seven presents two case studies illustrating the general approach adopted in drawing up the manpower aspects within the 1978-79 round of strategic planning at the Trent and Wessex RHA level. A brief overview of experience in other English Regions is also included. The spotlight turns in Chapter Eight to the role of the Area and District levels in manpower planning with the aid of an analysis of recent survey findings of current manpower practice. Attention is also given to future prospects in this field.

The discussion concludes in Chapter Nine with a review of the main themes and problem areas elaborated in the preceding chapters of the book. It concentrates on the interrelationship between the planning process and manpower management. The potential contribution which managers at all levels of the service can make is emphasised. The argument returns to explore the form which a more positive approach to manpower planning called for by the Royal Commission on the NHS might assume. (43)

NOTES

(1)   Royal Commission on the National Health Service, Report,
(Merrison Report), Cmnd. 7615, HMSO, London 1979, p.1.
(2)   Health and Social Service Journal, 30 March 1979, p.340.   Yet as
Enoch Powell, Minister of Health 1960-63, remarks, 'One of the most
striking features of the National Health Service is the continual
deafening chorus of complaint which rises day and night from every part
of it . . . The Universal Exchequer financing of the service endows
everyone providing it as well as using it with a vested interest in
denigrating it, so that it presents what must be the unique spectacle of
an undertaking that is run down by everyone engaged in it.'   J.E.
Powell, A New Look at Medicine and Politics, Pitman, London 1966, p.16.
(3)   H.Eckstein, The English Health Service, Harvard University Press,
Mass. 1970, Ch.1.
(4)   Evidence to Royal Commission, in Merrison Report, para.21.8.
(5)   Merrison Report, para.12.64;   and D.Clode, 'Circling the Pyramid by
Camel', Health and Social Service Journal, 3 August 1979, p.972.
(6)   I.Gough, 'State Expenditure in Advanced Capitalism', New Left
Review, no.92, 1975, pp.53-92;   Merrison Report, Table E6, p.431.
(7)   I.Gough, The Political Economy of the Welfare State, Macmillan,
London 1979, Ch.5.
(8)   Merrison Report, Table 3.8, p.23.
(9)   For contrasting views of state expenditure, contrast the interpretation of Ian Gough (notes 6 and 7 above) with, R.Bacon and W.Eltis,
Britain's Economic Problem: Too Few Producers, Macmillan, London 1976.
In the same vein, another commentator has described the NHS budget's
size as a 'major contributory factor' in Britain's current economic
difficulties - B.Watkin, The National Health Service: The First Phase,
Allen and Unwin, London 1978, p.159.
(10)   Resource Allocation Working Party (RAWP), Sharing Resources for
Health in England, HMSO, London 1976;   Merrison Report, especially Ch.2;
The Government's Expenditure Plans 1979-80 to 1982-83, Cmnd. 7439, HMSO,
London 1979, p.143.
(11)   Central Statistical Office, Annual Abstract of Statistics, HMSO,
London 1955 and 1978.
(12)   DHSS, Staffing of the National Health Service (England), DHSS,
London 1979, para.1.9.
(13)   Committee on Nursing, Report, (Briggs Report), Cmnd. 5115, HMSO,
London 1972.   General comments on aides and unqualified staff are
included in the Merrison Report, paras.12.36, 12.37, and Table 15.1.
(14)   T.Manson, 'Management, the Professions and the Unions', in
M.Stacey et al. (eds), Health and the Division of Labour, Croom Helm,
London 1977, pp.196-216.
(15)   J.Perrin, Management of Financial Resources in the National Health
Service, Royal Commission on the NHS, Research Paper no.2, HMSO, London
1978.
(16)   Merrison Report, para.12.27;   and also the evidence of the
Institute of Health Service Administrators in the Merrison Report,
para.12.29.
(17)   H.A.Clegg and T.E.Chester, Wage Policy and the Health Services,
Blackwell, Oxford 1957;   Merrison Report, Ch.12.
(18)   Financial Times, 5 August 1979.
(19)   Eckstein, The English Health Service, Ch.1.
(20)   Merrison Report, para.20.4.   For other views on reorganisation:
R.Brown, 'Structure and Local Policy Making in the Reorganised National

Health Service', <u>Public Administration Bulletin</u>, no.20, April 1976, pp.9-19; R.Levitt, <u>The Reorganised National Health Service</u>, Croom Helm, London 1976.

(21) Committee on the Senior Nursing Structure, <u>Report</u>, (Salmon Report), HMSO, London 1966; Committee on Local Authority and Allied Services, <u>Report</u>, (Seebohm Committee), HMSO, London 1968; Royal Commission on Local Government in England 1966-69, <u>Report</u>, Cmnd. 4040, HMSO, London 1969. Also important, <u>National Health Service Reorganisation: England</u>, Cmnd. 5055, HMSO, London 1972.

(22) House of Commons Expenditure Committee, <u>Eleventh Report</u>, vol.II, pt.1, HMSO, London 1977, p.381.

(23) RAWP, <u>Sharing Resources for Health in England</u>, para.1.2; for a critique of this document, Radical Statistics Health Group, 'A Critique of "Priorities for Health and Personel Social Services in England"', <u>International Journal of Health Services</u>, vol.8, no.2, 1978, pp.367-400.

(24) DHSS, <u>Priorities for Health and Personal Social Services in England</u>, HMSO, London 1976.

(25) <u>Merrison Report</u>, para.6.62.

(26) Clode, 'Circling the Pyramid by Camel'.

(27) L.Gunn and R.Mair, 'Staffing the National Health Service', in G.McLachlan (ed.), <u>Challenges for Change</u>, Nuffield Provincial Hospitals Trust, Oxford University Press, Oxford 1971, pp.263-295.

(28) R.Shegog, 'Manpower Research and the NHS', in G.McLachlan, B.Stocking and R.Shegog (eds), <u>Patterns for Uncertainty? Planning for the Greater Medical Profession</u>, Nuffield Provincial Hospitals Trust, Oxford University Press, Oxford 1979, p.211.

(29) The evidence of the Regional Administrators is reported without comment in the <u>Merrison Report</u>, 'The key to the deployment of manpower resources in the NHS is the redeployment of medical staff, for the necessary support in terms of other professional staff will follow providing the financial resources are likewise redeployed.' <u>Merrison Report</u>, para.12.58. For an excellent review of medical manpower planning see, A.Maynard and A.Walker, 'A critical survey of medical manpower planning in Britain', <u>Social and Economic Administration</u>, vol.11, no.1, 1977, pp.52-75. The same authors further explore this subject for the Royal Commission, A.Maynard and A.Walker, <u>Doctor Manpower 1975-2000</u>, Royal Commission on the NHS, Research Paper no.4, HMSO, London 1978. The official view is contained in, DHSS, <u>Medical Manpower - The Next Twenty Years, A Discussion Paper</u>, HMSO, London 1978.

(30) <u>Briggs Report</u>; DHSS, <u>Staffing of the National Health Service (England)</u>; and <u>Merrison Report</u>, Ch.13.

(31) Watkin, <u>The National Health Service</u>, Ch.3; L.Gunn and R.Mair, 'Staffing the National Health Service'.

(32) National Board for Prices and Incomes, <u>Pay of Nurses and Midwives in the National Health Service</u>, Report no.60, HMSO, London 1968; and <u>The Pay and Conditions of Manual Workers in Local Authorities, the National Health Service, Gas and Water Supply</u>, Report no.29, HMSO, London 1967.

(33) Maynard and Walker, 'A critical survey of medical manpower planning in Britain'.

(34) Discussed by several of the contributors in, G.McLachlan et al. (eds), <u>Patterns for Uncertainty?</u>; and A.Mejia, 'Migration of Physicians and Nurses: A World Wide Picture', <u>International Journal of Epidemiology</u>, vol.7, no.3, 1978, pp.207-215.

(35) <u>Merrison Report</u>, para.12.57. Nevertheless manpower forecasts do generate a not inconsiderable advantage for policy makers by their

apparent 'neutrality', and the specific character of predictions tends
to narrow the range within which decisions must be made.   'Undoubtedly
this is the secret of the abiding appeal of manpower forecasting to
governments.'   M.Blaug, 'The Uses and Abuses of Manpower Planning',
New Society, 31 July 1975, pp.247-248.

(36)   Civil Service Department, A Management Guide to Manpower Planning
Models, Civil Service Department, London 1975.
(37)   Scottish Home and Health Department (SHHD), Nursing Manpower
Planning Reports, nos.1-4, SHHD, Edinburgh 1974-5;   DHSS, National Staff
Committee for Administrative and Clerical Staff, The Recruitment and
Career Development of Administrators, (Hoare Report), DHSS, London 1978.
(38)   Merrison Report, para.13.4.
(39)   M.Kogan, The Working of the National Health Service, Royal
Commission on the NHS, Research Paper no.1, HMSO, London 1978, p.231.
(40)   Merrison Report, para.20.6.
(41)   Ibid., Appendix H.
(42)   Royal Commission on the National Health Service, The Task of the
Commission, HMSO, London 1976, para.8;   these points are further
developed in the Merrison Report itself, especially Ch.20.
(43)   Merrison Report, para.12.64.   Further suggestions on the role of
the DHSS and the NHS tiers are contained in the Consultative Document on
the restructuring of the NHS;   DHSS, Patients First, HMSO, London 1979.

2 Concepts and Problems

A. F. Long and G. Mercer

ISSUES IN MANPOWER PLANNING

To understand the state of manpower planning in the NHS, it is
necessary to locate the overall process of matching supply and demand in
its organisational context, specifically the NHS Planning System. The
discussion will be a preliminary to the more detailed analyses of
thinking and practice which are contained in subsequent chapters.

As the NHS was set up to provide a comprehensive health service,
manpower planning is charged with the responsibility of channeling the
most appropriate combination of staff skills to attain that goal within
available resources. This strikes at the qualitative heart of the
health service, since it determines how well the health of the
population is protected. It is perhaps lost when applying the textbook
definition of manpower planning as, 'a strategy for the acquisition,
utilisation, improvement and preservation of the enterprise's human
resources', (1) to the NHS. Health service growth has not been without
its difficulties in the past, and its future looks even more problematic. This reinforces the view that manpower planning should not be
carried out in a vacuum with total disregard for wider forces and
constraints.

A stylised representation of the manpower planning process is
illustrated in Figure 2.1. (2) The basic principle is to derive a
manpower plan that balances supply and demand requirements in tune with
overall corporate objectives. A forecast of manpower supply
encompasses an evaluation of existing resources and an assessment of
probable changes in that stock over the duration of service plans
through such processes as internal and external recruitment, levels of
labour turnover, impending changes in hours and conditions and other
external supply influences. Manpower demand is derived from the
intended type and level of health services. These supply and demand
forecasts must be satisfactorily matched before effective manpower
policies are written into the overall manpower plan for the organisation. The objective is to establish staff of the desired skills, in
the right place and at the intended time within the period covered by
the plan. Once a manpower plan has been devised and converted into
policies, it remains to monitor the progress and utilisation of

Fig 2·1 Overview of the Manpower Planning Process

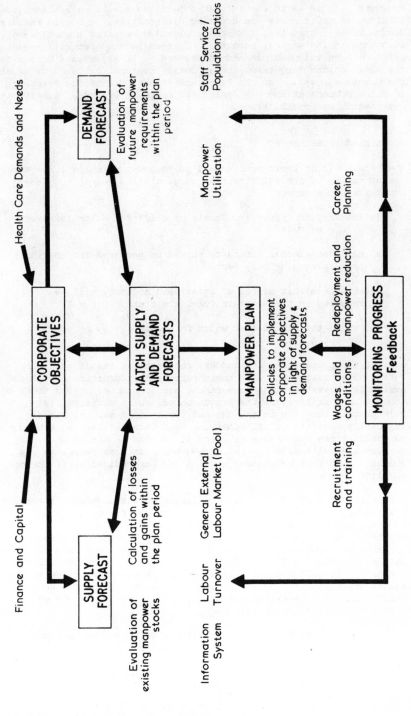

manpower. This is to ensure that objectives are being achieved, and if problems or new factors are creating difficulties, to enable remedial action to be instituted. Manpower planning requires a continuing feedback between its several aspects. Changes in one area will invariably react back on calculations made elsewhere. It may entail action over the short or the long term, and at local, regional or national levels. The day-to-day skills of the line manager are part of the manpower planning process as much as designated manpower officers, albeit with contrasting responsibilities.

PROBLEMS OF FORECASTING

The Department of Employment manual on manpower planning lists several issues worthy of special attention in generating supply and demand forecasts for manpower:

'1. identify the types and levels of skill for which forecasts should be made;

2. consider whether forecasts should be prepared for the whole organisation or only part;

3. establish what degree of detail and accuracy will be required in the manpower forecasts; and

4. decide the period over which forecasts should be attempted.' (3)

Since the preparation of manpower forecasts is itself a labour intensive activity, and with basic personnel information not always available, investigations have rarely been conducted beyond those groups thought most critical in the provision of health services. (4)   The bulk of the attention in the NHS has focussed on medical staff, especially hospital practitioners. Even these studies have been slow to consider the uneven distribution of doctors in the country, or between specialisms. (5)   As the NHS has felt less secure in its ability to attract sufficient nursing and paramedical staff the manpower spotlight has widened.

Consideration of staff groups in isolation has provoked increasing criticism. Health care requires a mix of staff - each with a specific contribution to make to the overall team effort. Flexibility in treatment regimes often requires that staff are correspondingly willing and able to substitute for other staff. (6)   Although this may be an attractive facility for manpower planning if supply and demand for labour are to gell easily it constitutes a hornet's nest for industrial relations. Despite the attraction of this integration of service and staff planning interpretations of how this should be developed in forecasting remain unexplored.

The size and geographical spread of the NHS have been major barriers in providing an even distribution of manpower across the country. Manpower forecasts need to be broken down to a Regional, if not more local level. The exact field of reference for recruitment has to be related to contrasting labour markets between staff. The existence of a small private sector for medical, nursing and several paramedical groups is the main dent in the NHS's monopolistic position as the provider of health care and buyer of health manpower. There is rather more concern about the international migration of staff - particularly medical. Forecasts of these flows into and out of the country have not proven very accurate in the past, with disruptive consequences for both medical education and the supply of staff. (7) Labour mobility of other employees, including administrative and clerical, works and ancillary staff, between the NHS and other sectors of the economy suffers from few barriers. In consequence, local managers have been left to recruit in these groups as appropriate. The estimation of manpower supply and demand has therefore been left in abeyance. The Royal Commission voiced the opinion that a central planning body along the lines of the Central Manpower Committee for Doctors and Dentists might be formed with a general forecasting responsibility, even though this runs counter to their anti centralisation theme. (8)

These issues also relate to the level of accuracy demanded in manpower forecasts. The margin of error is expected to diminish as the total workforce is broken down according to skill or grade within occupational categories, or if forecasts are made for different parts of the organisation across the country. Conversely, forecasting becomes more hazardous as the time span involved increases. The need for accuracy is highlighted in the health service because of the long periods of education and training through which a significant section of employees pass before becoming eligible to practise their professional skills. Not only is it necessary to plan several years ahead, but mistakes in determining the number and type of staff required will be extremely costly in terms of human resources and disruptive of health care provision.

An illustration of the manner in which forecasting over an extended time period has come to grief arises in medical planning. On the demand side, changes have occurred because of the movements in the birth rate, as well as uncertainties about the country's ability to maintain, let alone increase, health service funding. Supply has most obviously been confounded by fluctuating levels of migration. NHS manpower forecasts are further sensitive to turnabouts in the participation rate of groups which figure prominently in its workforce, especially women and part time staff. (9) One response has been to demand a more flexible data base so that, for example, the updating is carried out more frequently than the typical annual check. In addition, forecasters are encouraged to operate with more than one set of assumptions about crucial factors in the supply and demand equation such as labour turnover, migration and female participation rate. The intention is to provide more regular revision of forecasts, on a 'rolling' basis, while maintaining a long term perspective.

THE NHS PLANNING SYSTEM

The organisational context for health service manpower planning was restructured in 1976 with the establishment of the 'NHS Planning System'. (10) *Inter alia*, this sought to formalise the place of manpower within overall health planning. This integration reflected the corporate management philosophy encouraged in the NHS. If the traditional pattern of administration was a segmental structure, the corporate approach engendered a deliberately co-ordinated programme. No longer was manpower planning to be carried on by individual or local initiatives alone; rather had it become an organisational objective. The former structure was damned for its inefficiency, because it discouraged any measurement of overall performance and frustrated proper assessment of objectives or the monitoring of services. In contrast, these features were seen as the strengths of corporate planning. The latter was described as comprehensive, continuing, and formally applied. (11)

While defined as a total process, corporate planning encompasses short and long term aims. However, the dividing line between these has been left to individual organisations to determine in line with their own requirements. In the NHS, where capital schemes often take ten years or more to develop, and where the training of doctors extends over a similar period, there must be a long term time span that will permit planning across such crucial areas. The distinction chosen is between long term, strategic planning by care group which specifies the level of service provision over the next ten years, and operational plans. The latter cover no more than three years ahead and concentrate on the need to make the most out of existing facilities. Within this framework, a further possibility is project planning which concentrates on specific capital investments or equivalent policy decisions.

It was hoped that this system would both set the NHS on route for clear objectives, as well as introducing flexibility into planning. Since governmental pressures and turnarounds in the health field are not unknown this facility was regarded as essential for the NHS. Continual updating is instituted by moving plans forward on a 'rolling' basis. As each year covered by an operational plan ends, another is added; while strategic plans are worked out every four years as well as being rolled forward annually.

With this distinction between types of plan, the initiation of the whole planning cycle unfolds in the planning manual through four questions that structure the planning agenda: 'Where are we now?', 'Where do we want to be?', 'How do we get there?', and 'How are we doing?' (12) These points underlie the manpower planning process represented in Figure 2.1. Across the national, regional, area and district levels guidelines on policies, priorities and resources are communicated from higher to lower authorities. In turn, plans are fed back; and the procedure continues until realistic corporate plans are formulated which take appropriate note of health aims and constraints. In specifically manpower terms the key problem is to balance supply and demand forecasts, and to prepare policies as appropriate. The regular monitoring of progress is intended to maintain the plan on course, or at least in relative equilibrium.

The strategic plan comprises both interim and ultimate aims, including, 'results to be achieved (benefits to the patient or the community); levels of service to be provided (in terms of quantity or quality); changes in service patterns; or particular developments (or stages of developments) to be undertaken.' (13) As not all objectives carry equal weight or are equally attainable, the DHSS manual suggests that each be given a priority rating. There is a further recommendation that aims are framed in terms of service targets, and possibly the unit costs. Comments must be included on the implications for manpower supply and demand.

The first submission of strategic plans in 1977 uncovered a range of difficulties, and commitment from the Regions. It was therefore decided to repeat the whole exercise for submission to the DHSS in early 1979. Problems coalesced on a proper linking of service objectives to manpower, capital and revenue constraints. (14) Authorities found especial difficulty in estimating the revenue costs and manpower needs of specific schemes. Since the quantitative criteria in plan components were not heeded it was not possible to determine what constituted 'good' strategies along the lines envisaged by the DHSS.

There were further doubts about the restrictions imposed by the long and short term spans for planning. The upper limit did not always provide the necessary scope to plan for the desired balance of services. At the other end of the time scale, 'it is only when plans are approach-in an operational point, say three to five years away, that resource availability becomes crucial.' (15) An associated risk is that strategic and operational planning become wholly separate spheres of activity - a fear perhaps encouraged by the contrasting time periods covered and the designation of different responsibilities to the various tiers in the service. In comparison with the heady world of strategic planning, its operational counterpart can seem quite mundane. The DHSS manual speaks of a process which is interlocking, or a continuum, where short and long term plans feed into, as well as off each other. The supposition is that operational plans while prone to piecemeal engineering will also inform the longer strategy in terms of needs, priorities and general effectiveness.

In a complex organisation such as the NHS, with many levels of administration and jealously guarded professional autonomy, the balance of central and local control remains a contentious issue - as it had been before reorganisation. For while the centre retains strategic direction and control, and has instituted a formal system of monitoring performance, the claim is that there had been a meaningful decentralisation of decision making. The official documents talk of, 'real delegation downwards accompanied by accountability upwards.' (16) The system is not represented as hierarchical, but as one which is iterative between and within tiers.

Of course, no planning manual can be expected to provide easy solutions to all the problems which arise, and some latitude for manoeuvre is essential, but the NHS planning system provides the key parameter for the organisational context for health manpower planning. What requires investigation is how far in practice the quality of planning has been affected. In particular, have strategic and operational planning provided for a realistic manpower component? Is the service 'thinking manpower' as intended, and at all levels of the service? Clearly this entails understanding the planning context as well as the more specifically manpower issues of supply and demand.

SUPPLY OF LABOUR

In a typical representation the supply of labour has two facets.
Firstly, it starts from an evaluation of the existing manpower stock,
which is complemented, secondly, by calculation of losses and gains of
labour - including the pool of potential labour. (See Figure 2.1)   A
valid and reliable personnel information system on the retention,
recruitment and depletion trends is invaluable in this context.

Within the labour pool it is profitable to distinguish between a
group actively searching for employment, and another sector of persons,
either not currently working or employed outside of the health service,
but who nevertheless comprise potential recruits.   (See Figure 2.2)
The Briggs Report on Nursing contained figures which indicated that
among qualified nurses over 25 years of age the participation rate in
the NHS dropped substantially to approximately 50 per cent of the total
pool of trained staff.   This indicates a large pool of already trained
staff, who even if not actively looking for work, constitute a
reservoir of potential talent from which the NHS might draw. (17)   It
is among paramedical groups that the opportunities for employment
outside of the NHS are most significant and it is often argued that
efforts should be concentrated on trying to bring qualified chiropodists
and occupational therapists, for example, into a service sadly short of
their skills. (18)   A strong argument in the present economic climate
for the increased exploitation of this latent supply is that qualified
staff are obtained both more quickly and cheaply since there is no need
to resort to training new personnel from scratch.

Health service planning has been heavily criticised as overly capital
led, with manpower very much an afterthought.   There are instances of
hospitals being built only to function at less than capacity because
the full range of staff required are just not available. (19)   Hence
the rationale for conducting labour market surveys that will detail such
factors as local unemployment, competition for different sorts of
labour, housing and transport facilities.   Nationally, there are
further confounding factors, such as EEC directives, changes in the
working week, population changes, raising of the school leaving age, and
a change in the number carrying on to higher education.   In sum,
information is required on the size of gains and losses to the current
stock of manpower, as is in addition material on the pool of labour, in
all its forms, and the likely level of flow between these sectors.
Some of the key components in the supply of health manpower are
illustrated in Figure 2.2.   The unit of analysis can be any level of
authority within the service, although if lower than the national, it
would be valuable to distinguish a further source of gain to the current
stock which would come in the form of employees recruited directly from
another NHS authority.

A personnel information system that will provide a quick, accurate
snapshot of the workforce, as it is at present and as it is likely to
change in the planning period, is the basis for supply calculations.
The introduction of the NHS Planning System has given a significant
impetus to the collection of a basic minimum of manpower information.
Health authorities are required to submit a series of tables for the
Summary Analysis of Strategic Plans (SASP).   Data are required on
existing staffing and supply, together with turnover projections among

Fig 2·2 Components of Supply of Labour
(Freely adapted from: T. Hall, 'Supply' in T. Hall & A. Mejia, (eds) Health Manpower Planning. p92)

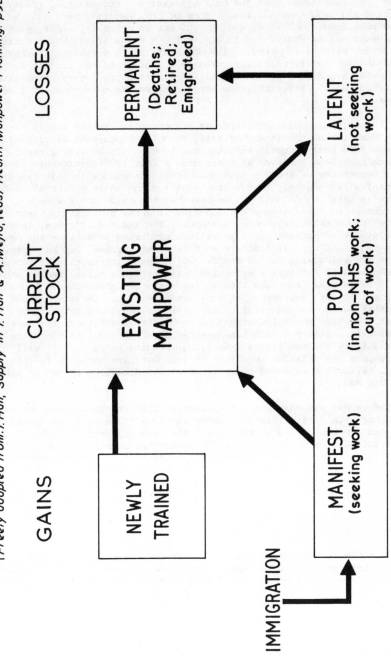

23

certain staff groupings as relevant to service provision.   Other
initiatives in personnel data collection concentrate on such areas as:
personal characteristics of employees - age and sex, relevant training
and qualifications;   and job characteristics - for example, grade, hours
worked and length of service.   Some of this material need only be
recorded once, such as date of birth, but in other instances, such as
occupational category, length of service and qualifications, continual
updating will be required.   The objective is to establish a personnel
information system which will provide a profile of the current workforce
as well as indicate potential crisis points in the future;   for example,
how many of a particular grade are due to retire over the next five
years.

   The projection of past trends as a forecast of future supply has
obvious limitations in a constantly changing employment situation.
There have been frequent exhortations to managers to keep a regular
check on labour turnover in their area - that is, recruitment, retention
and departures of staff - although current knowledge in this field still
contains large gaps.   Yet mistakes on a grand scale can be avoided if
care is taken to maintain up-to-date records, and to pay especial
attention to those groups and individuals whose stability pattern is
known to be relatively more variable.   The individual's age, length of
employment in current post, as well as expressed preference for mobility
between posts can all indicate what level of turnover may be expected
from a particular group of staff. (20)   Sound information on labour
turnover will facilitate effective policies for external recruitment as
well as internal supplies through transfers and promotion.   And in the
context of the restriction of services it will aid decisions about
whether forced redundancies rather than a planned reduction in the
workforce via 'natural wastage' or restricted recruitment are necessary.
A significant step beyond the measurement of turnover is therefore to
investigate the conditions underlying changing rates.   This will
encompass the relative impact of various work and non-work factors;   and
will be further enhanced by analysis of the direction of labour mobility
in the NHS.

   The extent and character of managerial intervention deemed necessary
to cope with difficulties in labour supply will on occasion spread far
beyond the boundaries of the NHS.   Yet some apparently internal
initiatives, such as a decision to expand the numbers in professional
training, are often transformed from an hitherto technical exercise into
a complex, politically sensitive task, as a range of sectional interests
are involved. (21)   Exactly the same comment applies to the translation
of the demand for health care into a specific mix of health personnel.

DEMAND FOR LABOUR

In the NHS, the planning system was geared to impose a detailed cross-
check between service targets, revenue and manpower resources.   These
constraints on the demand for health care and manpower have been brought
forward as substitutes for the controlling mechanism of the market in
private medicine, or where the individual patient's ability to pay has
been eliminated as an index of demand.   NHS planning has been further
linked with the RAWP formula for distributing central funds to the
Regions.   This establishes a grand total within which authorities

determine objectives.   Against that framework, the task is to convert
corporate objectives into service targets and associated manpower
resources.   In a detailed survey Hall identified four main approaches
to medium and long term forecasting of demand for health manpower:
health needs, where estimates are made of the level of health services
required to promote 'good health';   service targets, where demand is
constrained by such factors as revenue and capital availability;   health
demands, which is derived from the actual use of services;   and
manpower/population ratios, which convert a population to be served with
a fixed number of staff, according to specified criteria. (22)   A
modification of Hall's model is presented in Figure 2.3.   This
indicates the interaction of the 'health needs' and 'health demands'
approaches and their resolution in the form of 'service targets'.
Once that step has been taken the calculation of required manpower
follows directly from the specification of the type and range of health
services to be provided.   In the manpower/population approach manpower
demand is derived directly from the application of manpower ratios on
the population to be served.   In fact, it is also often premissed on
an opinion that a ratio of, for example, one doctor per 2,000 people is
adequate for health care, but such considerations are not explicitly
incorporated into the manpower calculations.

Hall in addition provides a comprehensive summary of the advantages
and disadvantages of the various approaches. (23)   In the British case
much of the rhetoric associated with the establishment of the NHS
concentrated on the health needs viewpoint where care would be provided
on the basis of need rather than ability to pay or some social or
political reasons.   Estimates of appropriate quality and quantity in
health services are made difficult by the lack of consensus across
public, government and health professionals.   There have been
complaints that in practice needs have been overly dominated by a
medical view of health and illness, and initiatives have been taken to
include public and other professional views.   Without controls such an
approach might stimulate total health service growth beyond the ability
of the NHS or Exchequer to provide or pay for it.   An initial check of
services could stem from a calculation of health demands, or actual
utilisation of existing services.   The obvious risk is that existing
inequalities in health care and access to it will be perpetuated.   On
the positive side, this approach should ensure that future satisfaction
with services at least maintains current perceptions.

If health needs and demands comprise the starting points for a
detailed analysis of manpower requirements, current economic
circumstances ensure that health service targets will be severely
constrained by specifying priorities within the general ability to
deliver those services.   These targets must be translated into
specific facilities, such as hospitals, health centres, beds and kidney
machines.   The next step entails a conversion of those items into so
much manpower.

The failure to establish agreed criteria for such population/service-
staff ratios has been manifest, and the DHSS felt obliged to provide a
wide ranging review of existing norms relevant to these calculations.
(24)   Their document was at pains to emphasise that such norms must be
set against the specifically local context, and further warned of hidden
assumptions in their use.   For example, the 1972 Quirk Report on Speech

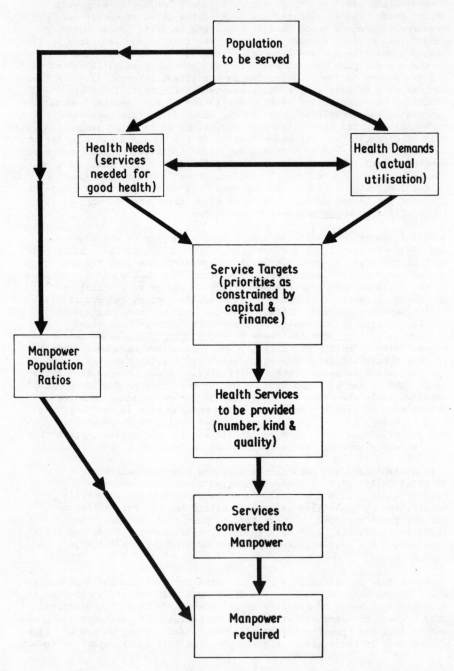

Fig 2·3 *Illustration of Approaches to the Estimation of Manpower Requirements.* *(Freely adapted from: T Hall & A Mejia (eds), Health Manpower Planning, p62)*

Therapy services suggested ratios applicable to such staff, but not all had appreciated that those ratios were predicated on the establishment of a grade of speech therapy helper. 'Non-establishment of this grade or poor recruitment to it would radically affect the estimated requirement for qualified speech therapists, and manpower planning on the basis of the quoted norms which did not take account of this factor would be inherently unsatisfactory.' (25)

An important element in the general pressure to adopt an increasingly cost-conscious approach in determining staff/service ratios has been the more effective utilisation of labour. 'Work study' approaches start from an analysis of the work process which measure the employee-hours per unit of production, and parallel 'productivity measurement' which fixes an output per employee hour. (26) Such approaches have made some inroads among ancillary staff while less frequently the work of health professionals is couched in such terms as nurses per bed, number of operations per surgeon, x-rays per radiographer. (27) Recently Maynard and Walker have argued forcefully that the traditional autonomy of doctors should be reconsidered, and the possibility admitted that it might be cost effective to substitute nursing time, for example, for doctor time in some areas of health care. (28)

Nevertheless measures of productivity are often notoriously difficult to compile, and potentially oblivious to the quality of health care. (29) Even if input time in terms of the number of employee hours is accepted, measures of output are constrained by the absence of a parallel yardstick of health – or the change effected. Instead proxy measures for quality control are substituted, such as the number of patients seen. Capital investment and technological innovations have stimulated similar controversy. For example, the hospital plans from the 1960s advocated the building of large, district general hospitals, partly because the concentration of services at one location was thought to improve the 'productivity' of the NHS – while enhancing patient care and reducing costs. The benefits now seem less certain. (30) Some improvements in technology have increased productivity – perhaps by 15 per cent in the case of the high speed drill in dentistry – but without comparable effect on the level of demand. Advances in heart surgery have sometimes reduced the number of patients treated, and greatly increased costs. (31)

The main alternative to estimating manpower demand represented in Figure 2.3 is based on manpower to population ratios. Such an approach has advantages in terms of the ease with which it is activated and interpreted. Furthermore, it provides a mechanism for maintaining the status quo, has clear applicability to an NHS which is relatively stable and has limited planning resources. That should not mask the ease with which unrealistic population to manpower ratios can be selected. In addition the use of these ratios in the NHS does not facilitate integrated manpower planning that focuses on a mix of staff or care groups rather than on single occupational categories.

The weakness of simple categorisations of health manpower planning in practice is graphically conveyed in an extract from the *Merrison Report* documenting the myriad influences requiring consideration when estimating demand for medical manpower:

'Some of the factors influencing demand for doctors are the birth
rate; the performance of the national economy (because
employment prospects for doctors depend, like those for the rest
of us, on money being available.to pay for them); the role of
doctors and their relationship with other health workers who may
undertake work which would otherwise be done by doctors;
developments in medicine; and changes in hours worked for
doctors. Health department policies may influence demand: for
example, the DHSS told us that the White Paper "Better Services
for the Mentally Ill" required 290 more consultants than at
present and something like 10 per cent more GPs would be
required to bring the average list size in England down to
2,000 patients. Charges such as these would depend on the
funds being available to pay for the doctors as much as there
being doctors available to employ.' (32)

SUMMARY

According to Mejia, central to the health manpower process are:
planning ('x health teams of y composition (are) in operation by time
t'); production ('x trained personnel of y type by time t'); and
management ('x units of service of specified quality delivered to a
defined population'). (33) The whole process is represented in more
detail in Figure 2.4. This amplifies the distinctions drawn in Figure
2.1, and in particular the matching of supply and demand forecasts, and
the manner in which these are brought into alignment within a manpower
plan as specific policies - all the time constrained by corporate
objectives. For if the manpower function is to make a meaningful contribution to health service provision and planning, it must be
integrated with other key components, namely capital and finance, and as
filtered through service targets, into the long term NHS strategy.

It was always recognised that the complexity and novelty of the new
NHS Planning System - not to mention manpower planning itself - would
mean that its early years would be especially testing. The planning,
production and management of resources have to be integrated into a
coherent and comprehensive system. Strategic planning in its infancy
has to determine an appropriate relationship between different authority
levels, and more specifically agree on the force and form of guidelines
issued.

It is also evident that 'thinking manpower' assumes a wide range of
questions about the demand for, and supply of, manpower; while the
injection of manpower within the planning process requires consideration
of an integrated approach which plans across care groups, or perhaps
across mixes of staff. This presumes both a sophisticated conceptual
approach to manpower planning that is fully supported by an adequate
information base, as well as a proper utilisation of the possibilities
offered within the organisational context for health planning. How
successful this period of innovation has been to date, and how the art
of manpower planning has developed, constitute the central themes
running through subsequent contributions to this book.

Overall Aim   To ensure the manpower needed by the health care delivery system

	Health Manpower Planning	Health Manpower Production	Health Manpower Management
Goal	To provide the framework within which the health manpower process takes place	To provide the manpower required	To optimise the use of health manpower
Objective	To specify the number of teams and the composition needed to improve the level of health up to a proposed level	To produce x people of y type	To determine manpower distribution and productivity standards, patterns of utilisation, and non labour inputs
Strategy	Regional planning and local programming. Health manpower project formulation. Aggregation, reconciliation and consolidation	Educational planning and programming educational objectives and teaching methods	Reorganisation: regionalisation; integration of prevention and cure; country health programming; primary health care; health manpower project management
Activities	Planning and programming Co-ordination Monitoring and evaluating implementation Research and Development	Recruitment campaign Definition of admission procedures and syllabus Definition of teaching methods Evaluation of process and products	Establishment and implementation of: supervision system; referral system; continuing education; recruitment and selection procedures; career development schemes; deployment of manpower; staffing patterns
Targets	x health teams of y composition in operation by time t	x trained personnel of y type by time t	x units of service of specified quality delivered to defined population coverage

Figure 2.4   The Scope of the Health Manpower Process*

*Source: A.Mejia, 'The Health Manpower Process', in T.Hall and A.Mejia (eds), Health Manpower Planning, p.36.

NOTES

(1)   Department of Employment, Company Manpower Planning, HMSO, London
1968, p.2; G.Stainer, Manpower Planning, Heinemann, London 1971.
(2)   Department of Employment, Company Manpower Planning, p.2.
(3)   Ibid., p.9.
(4)   Royal Commission on the National Health Service, Report, (Merrison
Report), Cmnd. 7615, HMSO, London 1979, para.12.58.
(5)   Merrison Report, Ch.14; A.Maynard and A.Walker, Doctor Manpower
1975-2000, Royal Commission on the NHS, Research Paper no.4, HMSO,
London 1978; DHSS, Medical Manpower - The Next Twenty Years, A
Discussion Paper, HMSO, London 1978.
(6)   Merrison Report, Ch.12, especially paras.12.26 to 12.35.
(7)   Ibid., Ch.14.
(8)   Ibid., especially paras.12.60, 12.26 to 12.35.
(9)   Department of Employment, 'Changing Composition of the Labour Force
1976-1991', Department of Employment Gazette, June 1979.
(10) DHSS, The NHS Planning System, HC(76)30, DHSS, London 1976.
(11) 'Corporate planning includes the setting of objectives to be
attained, motivating through the planning process and through the plans,
measuring performance and so controlling the progress of the plan, and
developing people through better decision making, clearer objectives,
more involvement, and awareness of progress.' D.Hussey, Corporate
Planning: Theory and Practice, Pergamon, Oxford 1974, p.6.
(12) DHSS, The NHS Planning System, p.8.
(13) Ibid., p.12.
(14) DHSS, 'Health Service Planning in England 1976-1978', DHSS, London
1979.
(15) R.Dearden, 'Why the Planning System is a good thing provided we
don't stick to the rules', Hospital and Health Services Review, October
1978, pp.345-346.
(16) National Health Service Reorganisation: England, Cmnd. 5055, HMSO,
London 1972.
(17) Committee on Nursing, Report, (Briggs Report), Cmnd. 5115, HMSO,
London 1972; J.Sadler and T.Whitworth, Reserves of Nurses, HMSO, London
1975; G.Lind, J.Luckman and C.Wiseman, 'Qualified Nurses Outwith the
Scottish NHS', Tavistock Institute of Human Relations, 1977.
(18) Merrison Report, Ch.15.
(19) B.Watkin, The National Health Service: The First Phase, Allen and
Unwin, London 1978, Ch.4.
(20) G.Mercer, The Employment of Nurses, Croom Helm, London 1979; M.J.
Nelson, 'The Market Place for Manpower', Southampton and South West
Hampshire Health District, Southampton 1977.
(21) See Chapter Five of this volume.
(22) T.Hall, 'Demand', in T.Hall and A.Mejia (eds), Health Manpower
Planning, World Health Organisation, Geneva 1978, Ch.3.
(23) Ibid., pp.82-83.
(24) DHSS, 'NHS Planning: The Use of Staffing Norms and Indicators for
Manpower Planning', DHSS letter from C.P.Goodale to Regional and Area
administrators, April 1978.
(25) Ibid., p.2.
(26) Department of Employment, Company Manpower Planning, pp.14-33;
Stainer, Manpower Planning.
(27) Merrison Report, Part III.
(28) A.Maynard and A.Walker, Doctor Manpower 1975-2000; DHSS, Medical
Manpower.

(29)   T.Baker, 'Productivity', in T.Hall and A.Mejia (eds), Health Manpower Planning, Ch.5; J.Rafferty (ed.), Health Manpower and Productivity, Heath, Lexington 1974.
(30)   B.Watkin, The National Health Service, Ch.4.
(31)   T.Baker, 'Productivity', pp.124-131.
(32)   Merrison Report, para.14.12.
(33)   A.Mejia, 'The Health Manpower Process', in T.Hall and A.Mejia (eds), Health Manpower Planning, p.36.

3 Case Studies of Manpower Planning

The three case studies included in this chapter provide examples of the way in which manpower planning across different NHS staff groups has been conducted.   Each study follows a common structure, providing an introduction to the problem area, a description of the methodology employed, an outline of some of the findings of the study, and concluding remarks.   The subjects of these case studies are medical staff within Wessex RHA, occupational therapists in Trent RHA, and nurses in the mental handicap specialty in West Midlands RHA.

The essential simplicity of approach required within manpower planning is well illustrated by these studies.   The intention is to provide examples of what might be undertaken by practitioners in the health field, both at the Regional and local level, by personnel and planning officers and managers themselves.   The discussion is extended to cover the implementation and outcome of these initiatives.   The methodologies presented are offered as examples of good practice.   Only through continued activity of this kind will the art of manpower planning be advanced.

MEDICAL MANPOWER PLANNING

P. Dixon

Introduction

Medical manpower planning has received significant attention,
particularly by the DHSS, since the inception of the Health Service in
1948. Much of the incentive for this attention is related to the
relationship between length of training and subsequent employment costs
with the desire, by careful planning, to ensure maximum utilisation of
the scarce resource. Medical manpower planning consequently had led to
a highly centralised control system (that is DHSS authorisation of new
posts in the consultant, senior registrar and registrar grades) the
justification for which must stem from a keen desire to reduce the risk
of under-utilising medical staff resources to run the services within
the NHS. As with any centralised control system there is an increase
in uncertainty at the local level where local planners and managers find
it very difficult to fit their medical staff planning into their
operational planning, because they have little control over the decision
on how many, grades and timing. This difficulty of planning and
scheduling medical staff often leads to frustration at the local level
and produces few incentives to plan the medical staff resource more
effectively. The typical result is the 'shopping list' approach which
is often adopted with the view that there will be a significant number
of items in the shopping list which are unlikely to be there when needed
(that is, in a given financial year) and that the final list may well be
near the finances available. A detailed analysis of each post is not
worth the effort and, in any case, one can always decide not to go ahead
with a post if more items become available than expected.

The purpose of this case study is to suggest an approach to medical
staff planning that can reduce the uncertainty felt at local level, yet
maintain some degree of control over the training and utilisation
aspects required at national level. This study is an attempt to
produce a ten year medical staff plan related to the demand for services
within the Wessex Region, which enables more involvement of medical
staff within the Region in determining their future staffing
requirements (consultation/participation), production of a framework for
future medical staff requirements which enables the Districts to plan
more effectively (planning), a positive policy on medical staff
investment (cash) to be developed at Regional and District level with an
accepted commitment by the authorities concerned (investment), and a
means of evaluating the effect on the Region of the DHSS control of
medical staff establishments (monitoring). Each of these aims will be
discussed in more depth towards the end of this case study after the
method has been described. It does, however, need to be borne in mind
that the above were key aims in the thinking that went into the
methodology.

Acknowledgement My thanks are due to Mrs. Audrey Bourne of the
Regional Statistics department, whose work on the population modelling
and programming aspects was invaluable.

Methodology

The Region decided, in view of the points mentioned in the introduction
concerning the involvement of medical staff and the need for a framework
for assessing future medical staff requirements, that a methodology more
related to the Regional needs ought to be developed. The current
literature on the subject, which is very clearly contained in the DHSS
discussion paper *Medical Manpower - The Next Twenty Years* (1) and in
McLachlan's book *Patterns for Uncertainty?* (2), tends to concentrate on
the characteristics of medical staff and the effect this has on the
supply of medical manpower and the career structure. The methodology
required in Wessex is almost totally orientated towards the medical
staffing requirements for the services to be provided within the Wessex
Region. In this way it is possible to start linking medical manpower
planning with the planning of capital and other revenue resources.

The method does not attempt to deal with the supply of medical staff.
It is felt that the supply questions are more properly the province of
the DHSS who are in a better position to develop central policy
regarding medical school intakes, legislation on immigration and
emigration, and the ability to guide the choice of curriculum of
university medical schools which influence the subsequent attitudes on
standards regarding the choice of specialty. All these above aspects
are outside of a Region's sphere of influence and have not been taken
into account in the development of the methodology described in this
chapter.

The methodology has therefore concentrated on medical manpower demand
forecasting. In doing this particular note needs to be taken of the
points raised in chapter four of the DHSS discussion paper on medical
manpower. (3) It identifies four specific factors that might affect
the number of doctors required in the future, namely: demographic
changes; reduction of existing geographical disparities; changes in
the organisation of medical practice; and improvement in the service
provided. The chapter considers the difficulties involved in carrying
out a forecast on the doctors required. When these difficulties are
examined in depth it becomes apparent that there is some benefit for a
Region in undertaking a manpower demand forecast as it is likely to be
more conversant with its particular demographic factors. It is also
much nearer the clinicians providing the service who are in possession
of the knowledge on possible changes in the organisation of medical
practice, and it is likely to know what improvement in services the
Region wishes to achieve.

The Wessex Region has for some time been at the lower end of the ratio
of medical staff to population when considering the levels of staffing
across Regions. In the past there has been a tendency to compare the
Region's medical staffing levels with the national level and to suggest
that additional staff are required within the Region to equal the
national levels. An assumption was made in developing the demand
forecast for medical staff in Wessex that, providing the local view was
that there were sufficient medical staff within the Region to provide a
particular service, then increases above the existing level should be
based on demographic or technical or organisational changes rather than
arbitrarily increasing levels to match the national or any other
Regional level. Consequently the Region has not attempted to examine

its position in relationship to other Regions or concerned itself with inter-regional disparities which have been of concern to the DHSS in its own medical manpower planning.

The method adopted within Wessex takes account of demographic factors, changes in the organisation of medical practice, and changes in the services provided. Before describing the method it is useful to consider what uses are to be made from the application of the method. By considering the uses to be made of the output it is easier to decide the type of classification of data that should be used in the development of the methodology. The reason for this can be linked back to the aims of the case study of consultation/participation, planning, investment, monitoring and implementation. If the results of the case study cannot be readily assimilated into these existing systems then much of relevance will be lost.

If one is to consult with medical staff about changes in medical practice, technological change, and so on, then one must talk in terms of specialties. These specialties must be capable of being divided or amalgamated into identifiable care groups (for example, acute, geriatric, psychiatric, maternity) if the Regional/Area planners are to relate the results to their service and capital plans. Local plans need to be District based, therefore the method should allow Districts to evaluate the consequences for their own District.

Medical staff need to be divided up into grades as there is so much pressure within the NHS to change the balance between grades, thereby producing a more equitable career structure. Also the centralised medical establishment control systems operate differently for each grade. For example, the control on the consultant grade primarily limits the allocation of new posts to Regions in the shortage specialties, that is, geriatrics, radiology and anaesthetics, whereas the control system on registrars and senior registrars tends to limit and in many cases freeze the creation of any new posts in more attractive specialties such as general medicine, general surgery, obstetrics and gynaecology. It also attempts to redistribute posts in the registrar and senior registrar grades between Regions by withdrawing the approval for posts from the more well off Regions.

The work of hospital medical staff is generated from the population. This bald statement hides several underlying organisational factors, namely: the work of non-consultant grades is determined by the consultant; only the consultant can take on new patients, thereby determining the total caseload. This is complicated by the extent of emergency work, for example in accident and emergency services which may vary from District to District, and for the work of anaesthetists, radiologists and pathologists which is largely determined by other clinicians. Given these organisational factors the method developed makes a distinction between consultants and other medical staff (including clinical assistants, GPs) and within consultants between anaesthetics, pathology and radiology consultants and clinical consultants. Only those (consultants) to whom patients are referred directly by the GP are actually related to demographic factors.

The method starts with the population as shown in Figure 3.1. There is much discussion within all Regions on whether one should plan to a

Fig 3·1 *Derivation of 1988 Consultant Sessions*

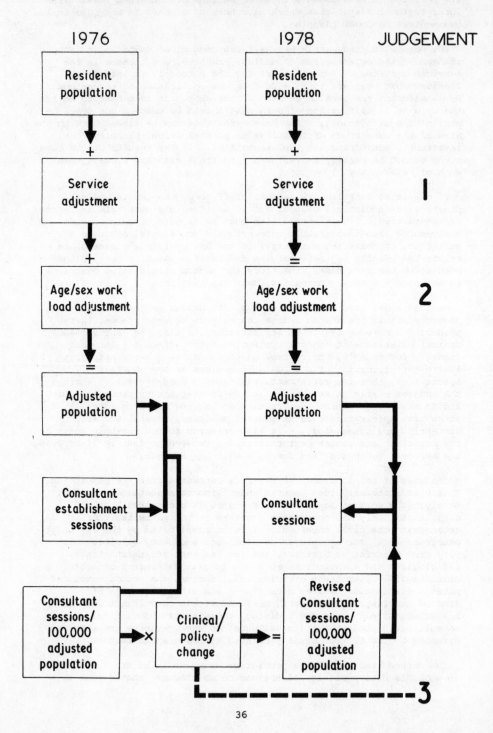

1976	1978	JUDGEMENT

Resident population → + → Service adjustment → + → Age/sex work load adjustment → = → Adjusted population

Resident population → + → Service adjustment → = → Age/sex work load adjustment → = → Adjusted population

1

2

Consultant establishment sessions

Consultant sessions

Consultant sessions/ 100,000 adjusted population → × → Clinical/ policy change → = → Revised Consultant sessions/ 100,000 adjusted population

3

resident population or to a catchment/service population. Some of the differences of these catchment populations from a resident population are due to the availability of resources in a given District. If these resources are put right then it may well be that a change in the GP referral of patients could ensue. As is well known, however well provided a District may be with resources, this still does not prevent individual GPs from referring patients to Districts outside of their resident population area. In considering planning for ten years hence a view needs to be made on whether a given specialty catchment area is likely to change because of changes in the availability of resources. Underlying factors such as travel routes, clinical preferences of GPs, and changes in resources will affect the judgement on the scale of change. The method shown in Figure 3.1 measures the weighting of the resident population of the District required to determine its service population and the view taken of the changes over a period of time. This is called Judgement Point 1.

There has been a tendency in the past to plan future medical staff on the basis of a straight ratio of consultant sessions to population. Such a method is not sensitive enough. It is necessary to take into account the age and sex structure of the population, particularly in specialties where the workload varies considerably according to age and sex. If all Districts had the same age/sex structure there would be no need to worry about the workload thrown up by individual age and sex groups. However, many Districts deviate quite considerably from the national population pattern. This is particularly so in the Wessex Region where the south coast has an extremely high percentage of its population in the over 65 age group. The following example is inserted to show the effect one of the factors, age, can have on the level of consultant staffing required in two totally different Districts.

District A's population is 400,000 and produces, in specialty X, 2,000 cases in one year. 1,000 of these cases are aged over 65. Supposing there are twenty consultant sessions in the District and that 10 per cent of the population is aged over 65, how many consultant sessions would be needed for the same size population in District B with 20 per cent of its population aged over 65? The figures and calculations can be seen in Table 3.1 (see p.38). In other words, the number of consultant sessions required for District B's population is calculated on the basis of the rates of cases to population in District A. The first step is to obtain the expected number of cases arising for the population aged over 65 and 65 or less. Then the total number of (age-weighted) cases are found. The number of consultant sessions required is calculated by applying the rate of consultant sessions to cases in District A to the expected number of (age-weighted) cases in District B. So, in District B nine additional sessions are required, equalling almost one whole-time equivalent consultant.

If an age-weighted approach was not adopted both District A and B would expect the same number of cases. In other words, the rate of cases to the population, ignoring age, would be equal to five per 1,000. Taking age into consideration, the age-weighted rates are in fact five per 1,000 for District A and 7.2 for District B. Admittedly few population structures have such extremes but this hypothetical situation demonstrates the need to weight the population according to the cases thrown up in a given specialty by the particular age/sex structure of that population.

Table 3.1
Age-weighted Populations

	District A[a]	District B[b]
District Population	400,000	400,000
Population aged over 65	40,000	80,000
Cases aged over 65	1,000	$\frac{2.5}{1000}$ x 80,000 = 2,000
Cases per 1,000 population aged over 65	2.5	2.5
Cases aged 65 or less	1,000	$\frac{0.28}{1000}$ x 320,000 = 890
Cases per 1,000 population aged 65 or less	0.28	0.28
Total Cases Age-weighted	2,000	2,890
Consultant Sessions	20	29
Consultant Sessions per case	0.01	0.01

Notes

[a] Figures for District A are given.

[b] Figures for District B, other than those on the population base, are expectations, arrived at by applying the appropriate rate of cases to population in District A to the population of District B.

The data used for the method in Wessex to weight the population for age and sex in relation to workload was that contained in the Hospital In-patient Enquiry data available nationally. Clearly the pattern of take-up of cases in a given age/sex can change. The most obvious example in recent years is the dramatic decrease in the treatment of tonsils and adenoids in ENT in the 5-14 age group. A judgement can be made on the direction and size of these changes by the profession and these can be built into a forecast. Therefore the method should contain a weighting of a District's population for its age/sex workload factor which can be changed for future forecasts (Judgement 2, see Figure 3.1).

The DHSS discussion document on medical manpower suggests some of the factors affecting change are: the shift in emphasis from hospital to community care; the possibility of having relatively more consultants than juniors; some redistribution of work between medical and non-medical staff; the effects of technological change; and a shorter working week. (4) These are just some of the factors, there may well be more. It is assumed that all these factors are not population linked and that they are more likely to change the level of consultant sessions to population (age-weighted).

This is the most difficult area to quantify and yet it should not be ducked just because it is difficult. It has already proved possible in Wessex to ask a group of doctors what changes are likely to occur in the ratio of consultant sessions/weighted population. Often they have a feel of the actual number of doctors or sessions involved rather than a percentage figure. By trial and error it is possible to work back to a percentage and thus relate it to a consultant sessions/population rate. This judgement is termed, in the method, a clinical/policy judgement (Judgement 3, see Figure 3.1).

The DHSS document states that there are certain areas in which there is clear unmet demand at present, and where there are not enough doctors available to provide a 'service which the Health Authorities wish to provide'. (5)   These it lists as: the 'client groups' in the specialties of psychiatry, geriatrics and paediatrics, where there is a government policy of a higher rate of growth; and the 'support' specialties of anaesthetics, radiology and pathology, where a higher standard of medicine and new techniques have increased demand.   The same situation as that described above is involved; that is, the quantification of the level of change in the consultant sessions/ population for client groups and level of consultant sessions/other sessions in respect of support specialties.   These changes are incorporated into the clinical/policy judgement factor (Judgement 3, see Figure 3.1).

To summarise the approach, the resident population is adjusted to take account of patient flows (service adjustment) and the workload generated by a particular District's age/sex population structure when compared with the Wessex population structure in 1976.   The consultant sessions are related to the adjusted population to produce a ratio.   A judgement (clinical/policy change) is made on whether this ratio is likely to change by 1988 and a new ratio produced.   This new ratio is applied to the 1988 adjusted population to derive the number of consultant sessions required in 1988.

An adjustment factor is built into the Teaching District's figures of one-seventh to allow for teaching; for example, the consultant sessions required in 1988 times one-seventh.   This level was originally built in by the DHSS when the first medical staffing levels were agreed for the teaching district when it became a teaching hospital HMC.   A separate derivation of anaesthetic, radiology and pathology consultant sessions was undertaken by establishing a ratio between surgical and anaesthetic sessions and a ratio between surgical/ medical sessions and radiology or pathology sessions; making a judge-ment on whether this ratio should change by 1988; and then applying the new ratio to the sum of sessions derived for surgical or medical and surgical sessions above.   A separate derivation was also undertaken in respect of all the other grades of medical staff, for example, medical assistant, SHMO, senior registrar, registrar, SHO, HO, clinical assistant and hospital practitioner grade.   In brief this was done by examining the current ratio of the whole-time equivalents in each grade to the consultant whole-time equivalents by each specialty and making a judgement on whether a change was required in this ratio for the future. The new ratio for each grade was then applied to the consultant sessions derived for 1988 from Figure 3.1 thus generating the number of medical staff required in each grade by specialty.

Findings

As previously stated the increase in a front line specialty generates additional work for support specialties such as anaesthetics, pathology and radiology. Because of this there is a need when forecasting to relate support specialties to the total consultant sessions in selected front line specialties. Table 3.2 shows the total increases required between 1976/88 in consultant anaesthetic staffing just to keep the same ratio of anaesthetic sessions to total surgical sessions. The figure shows that approximately thirteen whole-time equivalent anaesthetists will be required and takes no account of any developments with anaesthetics such as pain clinics which may require a higher ratio of surgeons to anaesthetists in the future. Given that anaesthetics, pathology and radiology are shortage specialties (difficult to recruit to) at present, the ability of any Region to obtain the numbers involved could severely limit the ability to increase the numbers of staff in the front line specialties. This sort of conclusion will also affect the pace of building up of capital provision within the Region.

Table 3.2
Changes in Consultant Anaesthetic Sessions

	1976	1988	Changes from 1976
Surgical Sessions	2075	2464	389
Ratio of Surgeons/ Anaesthetists	2.6	2.6	0
Anaesthetic Sessions	798	948	150

The data can also be presented as shown in Table 3.3. This illustrates the sum of the changes required between 1976/88 in each grade for three specialties, together with the total for all specialties. These figures can be costed to give a District an illustration of the level of investment it requires per annum over the next decade. On this basis the District illustrated should be planning for at least one consultant per annum and the equivalent of two junior or other medical staff per annum.

Table 3.3
Change in Medical Staffing 1976-1988

	Cons. sess.	SHMO/ MA w.t.e.	Senior Reg. w.t.e.	Reg. w.t.e.	SHO w.t.e.	HO w.t.e.	CA/HPG w.t.e.
General Medicine	-8	-	+1.0	-	-	+2.5	-1.0
Geriatric Medicine	-2	-1.5	-	+0.5	+2.0	-	+2.0
Paediatrics	+8	-1.0	+0.5	+0.5	-	-	-

A third way of presenting data is by care group. Service planners require the number of medical staff by care group and area, not by specialty or grade. This requires a fair degree of rearrangement of the data but is nevertheless important in the evaluation of future ten year corporate/strategic planning. (6) Table 3.4 (see p.41) shows the data produced from the model.

Table 3.4
Total WTE Medical Staff by Care Group
(including Community Health Staff)
for the Region 1976-1988[a]

Care Group	1976	1988	% Change
Child	69	95	(38%)
Regional Services	110	149	(35%)
Community Care	292	378	(29%)
Elderly/Physically Handicapped	126	161	(28%)
Acute	968	1136	(17%)
Maternity	79	92	(16%)
Mental Illness	163	187	(15%)
Mental Handicap	19	18	(-5%)
HQ	49	55	(12%)
TOTAL	1875	2271	(21%)

Note

[a] Support medical staff are distributed across care groups

The final example is to show the data in terms of costs. The costs
at 1976 price of the projected increase over the next ten/twelve years
are shown in Table 3.5.   These can be discussed with treasurers as a
basis for recommending a medical staff investment programme.   This
programme determines the annual level of finance that needs to be
allocated for the annual medical staff programme.   This investment is
almost totally that required to keep pace with the population.
Consultation with the profession is likely to increase this level
probably to one around the 2 per cent per annum level as increases in
clinical workloads due to technological change are brought to
management's attention.

Table 3.5
Medical Staff Investment Programme

	1976	1988	% Change
Cost (£000s) at 1976 price levels	14,271	16,797	18%

The method also allows one to monitor annually medical staff
programmes agreed for each District; the rate of change in specialties;
and the level of investment actually incurred.   It is also important to
evaluate the potential change against central DHSS medical establishment
control policy.   Is the Region in line with DHSS career planning
policy?   Is the Region in line on house officer posts with the DHSS
recommended level of increase to cope with medical school output?   Is
the Region affected by central policy or regional redistribution?   Are
the Region's service plans affected by non-implementation of specific
posts at a particular time because of central control policy?

Conclusion

The above method suggests an approach that tries to forecast over the
next ten years medical staff requirements, by involvement of the staff

providing the service. It will take about two years to meet all
specialty groups and interested parties to formulate an agreed policy
within the Region. If this can be achieved it would pave the way to
bridging the gap between a centralised DHSS medical establishment
control system which tries to reduce the risk in bad planning of scarce
resources and the uncertainty that a centralised system produces at
local level. This uncertainty can be described as the inability to
plan a given medical staff post at a point in time when a particular
service is being developed within a District thereby jeopardising the
successful implementation of that particular service or even the opening
of a new building.

It is perhaps too much to hope that providing an agreed framework
within which a Region and its Districts/Areas can plan their medical
staff resources at a sensible pace could result in a devolution to local
level of the control of medical staffing change. An acceptance that
market forces can operate without detriment to the overall planning of
the supply of medical manpower which must ultimately rest at national
level would be required to devolve decision making to the extent
suggested. The reasoning behind this point is that if a District
advertises a post, in line with its own services, at the point in time
it is required it will not in the end seriously affect the distribution
of medical manpower between Regions or the career structure balance
within the NHS. It is an unwillingness to accept that free market
forces would not have such a catastrophic effect that perpetuates the
desire to rigidly control medical manpower at a national level. The
hypothesis within this paper suggests that a more constructive approach
to medical staff planning at Regional level would seem to facilitate a
possible future move in central control policy.

PLANNING THE PARAMEDICS: THE CASE OF OCCUPATIONAL THERAPY

M. Blunt

Introduction

This case study details the development of a basic methodology for
planning the paramedical groups of staff in the Trent Region.   The
methodology was developed through successive reports on different staff
groups and has been amended in each report to suit the particular
requirements of that group of staff.   This case study refers
particularly to the problems and requirements associated with the
planning of occupational therapists in the Region.   However, the basis
of the methodology is common to all the reports.   The studies on the
paramedical groups of staff arose from initial needs to answer
individual and specific pressing questions of policy.   In order to
answer such problems a full planning study, attempting to assess the
present position and future demand for and supply of the profession, had
to be put 'in train'.   This resulted in each case in recommendations
which have set the direction for training policy for the profession
within the Region over the next decade and beyond.

The study of occupational therapy arose from pressure within the
Region to open a further school of occupational therapy to add to the
one already in existence.   If such a policy were adopted it would have
a great effect on the future numbers of occupational therapists that
would become available for employment in the Region and nationally.
The Region's manpower planning section was set the task of identifying
the problems associated with such a policy and pointing towards
remedies.

Trent is a health service region at present deprived of resources on
most measures;   financial, buildings, equipment and manpower.   Present
policies to redistribute resources towards deprived regions would
therefore have a major effect on staffing numbers over the next decade.
The numbers of occupational therapists would need to grow rapidly over
the next decade if Trent was to meet its service targets.   However,
decisions on training schools, maximum intake levels to training,
standards and so on for paramedical staff are taken nationally by the
respective Colleges of the professions, serviced and aided by the
Council for Professions Supplementary to Medicine.   Thus, the need was
not only to convince policy makers within the Region, but to provide
them with sufficient facts and arguments to confront the decision takers
at national level, who weigh the interests of the NHS as a whole against
the specific interests of the profession.

Throughout the development of the paramedical group of studies some
major principles developed on the conduct of such studies.   These were
followed and further developed in the course of the analysis of

Acknowledgement   The author is indebted to those members of his staff
who actually carried through the work described above: Miss Laura
Noel, who was a main contributor to the original methodology for the
paramedical studies; and Mrs. Kath Drayton, author of the report on
occupational therapists.

occupational therapists. Firstly, the practical nature of the problem and the answers required was paramount. Therefore, the analysis had to be simple and the answers arrived at capable of being implemented as Regional policy. Secondly, limited time scales and resources demanded that information collection and analysis had to be kept to a minimum and would, therefore, not involve a survey of individual staff. Thirdly, both management and staff should be informed and involved in the study from its inception, as their co-operation in data collection, their ideas, their problems, their views and their professional expertise provided the backbone of the study. Fourthly, the fullest possible consultation had to be carried out before, during and most essentially after the study (but before policy was agreed). Results could then be tested by the severest critics: management, who finance and use the staff; and the profession, on whom the study was based. Thus, if the study was approved of after such rigorous consultation its validity and more important its acceptance both by management and the profession was assured. Policy makers could then be given a clear mandate from which to work.

Methodology

The development of a methodology through the series of studies of para-medical staff was perhaps the most crucial element in their success. The principles by which the studies were constrained demanded a simple yet comprehensive structure as well as one which would easily bring about an understanding of the main problems, policy questions and recommended answers in the eyes of the policy makers. To begin with the main elements of the staffing situation had to be identified. This would provide a structure to the analysis and allow an easier definition of information needs, analysis needs and subsequently the definition of present and future problems and possible solutions.

The basis of manpower planning being a question of demand and supply and the synthesis of these factors over time provided the key to the methodology. A structure for the reports developed as set out in Figure 3.2.

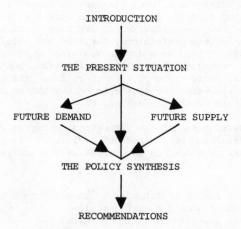

Figure 3.2   The Structure of the Paramedical Reports

An introduction described the main characteristics of the Region, its population and its major problems in the provision of health care services, the development and purpose of occupational therapy and the differing roles of staff in both NHS and local authority employment. The description of the present situation of occupational therapists in the Region and their problems comprised the first major element of analysis. Some of the data on which it was based were provided from computer or other statistical records. The majority of data, however, was obtained direct from District occupational therapists in the case of health service employees, and from Principal occupational therapists for local authority employees. Data on health service and local authority staff was shown and analysed separately. Table 3.6 (see p.46) sets out the analyses undertaken, their purpose, the methodology used in their presentation, and the sources of the data.

Future demand The analysis of future demand for staff was concerned with finding and utilising the best available methods of assessing the need for staff, firstly without entering in any detail the thorny and inconclusive area of staffing norms and secondly without adequate indications from health service Areas or local authorities of their future requirements. Figure 3.3 shows the analyses undertaken in attempting to assess future demand.

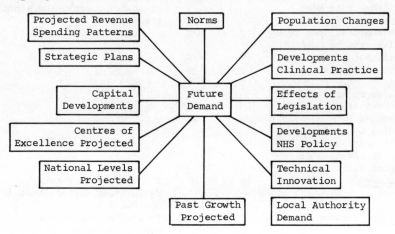

Figure 3.3   Future Demand - Analyses Undertaken

No widely acceptable staffing norms were available, but some discussion of local systems used by Head occupational therapists was entered into. These ranged from 'dependency' type calculations to calculations of numbers of patients and individual treatment times. However, none were of any real use in estimating future demand in a strategic planning context. Some discussion of general issues was undertaken, including likely population changes, developments in clinical practice, the effect of legislation, developments in health service policy and technological innovation. These were useful as general background and to set later work within its environmental context, but again were unable to be used to quantify future demand beyond showing the general direction of the profession as one of growth rather than one of contraction.

Table 3.6
The Present Situation - Analyses, Purposes, Presentation
and Data Sources

Analysis	Method[a]	Source[b]	Purpose
Current Staffing Position			To enumerate levels and
Numbers and whole-time			patterns of employment in
equivalents (wte)	T	C	the Region and basic
Organisation of staff and			differences in the compos-
their managerial units	O	X	ition of the workforce.
Numbers male and female	T	C	
Numbers full and part time	T	C	
Numbers married and single	T	M	
Age Structure			To judge different age group
All workforce	T/G	C	patterns brought about by
Full time staff	T/G	C	wastage - problems and
Part time staff	T/G	C	future retirement levels.
Staffing Structures and			To establish staffing
Shortfalls			shortfalls in detail and
Full time/Part time by			reasons for them, and
grade	T	C	analyse the different levels
Establishment/In post			of staffing provision within
comparison of areas			the Region.
with shortfall per cent	T	M/C	
Establishment to			
population	T	M/X	
In post to population by			
Area	T	C/X	
Vacancies by Area and as			
per cent of Regional			
vacancies	T	M	
Vacancies by Grade and			
Health Care Sector			
Grade distribution of			
in post staff			
Recruitment	O	M	To note the different
			recruitment difficulties in
			the Region.
Supporting Services	O	M/C	To analyse the effect of
			supporting services on
			staffing levels.
Clinical Placements	O	M	To note the situation of
During Training			clinical placements and
			their effect on staffing
			levels.
Turnover (over a two year			To analyse turnover rates
period)			and the flow of staff
Grade recruitment rate	T	M	around and in and out of
Grade wastage rate	T	C	the Region and the reasons
Origin of recruits	T	M	for them.
Reasons for leaving	T	M	
Flows into and out of			
Region	T	M	
Turnover by grade	T	M/C	

(See bottom of p.47 for Notes)

Past growth rates were analysed to provide some indication of future growth rates. National and Regional growth rates over the past 10 years were analysed (7) and a graph of staffing numbers was used to illustrate this. Using analyses published by the DHSS Manpower Intelligence Branch, on likely growth rates in staff over the next decade, national average staffing levels per 100,000 population were projected forward to 1988 and the numbers of staff Trent would require to meet that average were assessed. (8) The staffing levels of the best staffed Region were assessed and projected to 1988 as an indication of excellence in the practice of occupational therapy and Trent's requirement to meet such levels was noted. (9)

The number of occupational therapists needed in the hospital service being linked to the provision of the places in which they work, that is hospitals, consideration of future capital developments and their requirement for occupational therapists would therefore provide a good indication of future demand. Areas were contacted, major developments listed as to their proposed date of operation and the year of recruit- ment and levels of the occupational therapists needed were assessed by Area staff. At the time when the analysis was being undertaken only two of the eight strategic plans of the Trent Areas were available. An estimation of average growth rates was made from these and applied to other Areas to provide another indication of demand.

Future demand depends not only on the need for and supply of occupational therapy, but also on the finance available to pay for increased staffing levels. As a part of the preparation for the Regional strategic plan the manpower planning section had completed an analysis which looked at the way in which authorities spent their revenue monies on staff in 1976 and had projected this spending pattern on to revenue forecasts for 1988, thus creating an analysis which could state 'if you continue to spend your money in the same way as you did in 1976 you will buy these additional staff'. The figures thus produced for occupational therapists were used as a further indication of demand (or perhaps a possible constraint on demand). The different methods of assessing future demand each had their own particular strengths and weaknesses. The levels of increase required by 1988 ranged from a low of 73 per cent based on previous spending patterns to a high of 163 per cent based on capital developments. (10) The outcome was a compromise demand figure of an additional 180 occupational therapists. This entailed an increase of 116 per cent compared with an increase of 115 per cent in the last 10 years. (11)

Attempts at obtaining means of assessing future local authority demand for occupational therapists failed. As the profession itself thought

Notes for Table 3.6 (p.46)

a Method of presentation: O - Textual observations and numbers.
  T - Tabulated.
  G - Graphical representation, histogram, graph, and so on.

b Data source: C - Data held on computer records.
  M - Manual data obtained from managers.
  X - Others.

there would be little increase in the local authority centre it was
decided to utilise the existing 25 per cent in post shortfall from
establishment levels as the demand figure. (12)   The final 10 year
projection arrived at was agreed as an additional 200 posts.

Future supply   The analysis of present training arrangements and
estimation of the future supply of staff was intended to examine the
adequacy of present arrangements, to generally probe the workings of
the supply system, and from it to point towards changes or improvements
which would better meet the demand of the Region in the future.
Figure 3.4 shows the analyses undertaken in assessing training arrangements and the future supply of staff.

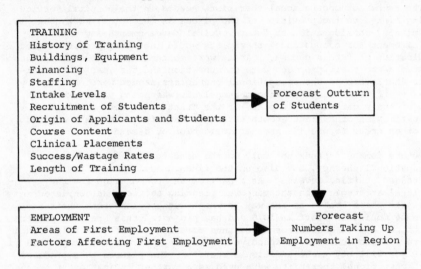

Figure 3.4   Future Supply - Analyses Undertaken

The history of occupational therapy training in Trent, its resources
in terms of buildings, equipment and staff and its financing, the
course content, syllabus, examination systems, clinical placements, and
success and wastage rates gave useful background against which the
effectiveness of the training school could be judged.   The levels of
student intake, method of recruiting students, the origin of applicants
and the eventual students selected (13) gave insights into the
operational policies of the training school.   A combination of the
analysis of intake levels, student wastage, and length of training
allowed a forecast of future outturn of students to be made over the 10
year period required.

An analysis of areas of first employment of students combined with
future forecasts of the number of students qualifying allowed a judgement to be made as to the number of students who under present policies
were likely to enter employment in the Trent Region.   Inspection of
the origins of students and the area of their clinical placements
against the areas in which they took up employment allowed judgements
to be made about the importance of these factors in the students'
initial choice of employment.

<u>Policy synthesis</u> The preceding analyses comprised the bulk of the consideration of the data collected. The task now was to take from that consideration the main strands of existing problems, future demand and existing supply and weave from it recommendations that through their incorporation into policy and action would seek to meet the needs of the Region for occupational therapists over the coming decade. This was accomplished through the analyses set out in Table 3.7.

Table 3.7
The Synthesis of Demand and Supply

Existing Staff

Plus Future Demand   = Net Numbers Required in Post

Plus Wastage over the Decade   = Net Numbers Required to Enter
                                      Employment

Minus Supply from Outside the   = Net Numbers Required from Training
         Region

Minus Projected Numbers   = Training Shortfall
         Qualifying in Trent

Plus Additional Wastage from   = Total Increase in Intake Required
        Training on Shortfall
        Number

   A consideration of the flows of experienced staff into and out of the Region led to conclusions regarding their net wastage and recruitment rates. Similar conclusions were arrived at for newly qualified staff. The way was then clear to produce a numerical synthesis of demand for and supply of staff in order to note future shortfalls or surpluses in each of the 10 years of the coming decade. Existing staff plus future demand produced desired future staffing levels. The addition of a figure for wastage over the period allowed a judgement of how many occupational therapists the Region would need to employ in order to achieve and maintain those levels. The analysis of flows of staff allowed consideration of the net staffing gains likely to be achieved from other Regions, and the subtraction of this from the net numbers required allowed a judgement of how many occupational therapists the Region itself would need to produce. The likely numbers entering employment in the Region from training in the Region set against the numbers it was now known the Region would need to produce allowed consideration of the present training shortfall. The shortfall comprised the additional number Trent needed to train in order to achieve the levels of staffing it desired. However, in order to arrive at a judgement of the intake to training required, an additional number had to be added in order to take account of wastage during training. Noting the increase in intake required, the alternative of expanding the present school or developing a new school for occupational therapy training was examined. (14)

Findings

From the initial analysis of the current staffing situation a large number of existing problems were defined that needed to be remedied in the future. The Region was one of the most understaffed for occupational therapists in the country. This situation was ameliorated by a higher than average employment of unqualified 'helpers' but this led to a dilution of the standard of service given. The profession was female dominated and the backbone of the service was provided by young and therefore relatively inexperienced staff. This also led to a large turnover level as women left to follow husbands' moves out of the Region, or left to become housewives or mothers. The average working life of an occupational therapist was less than seven years. Instability in the workforce was therefore a major factor which could be affected by greater use of part time staff and encouragements to staff to return to work after breaks in service.

Perhaps the most important single finding in the report was the disparity of staffing levels and problems within the Region largely brought about by the location of the training school and the school's operational policies. In the case of both NHS and local authority services the health authorities closest to the training school had the highest establishment levels, the highest in post levels, the lowest levels of vacancies, the best grade distribution patterns, the least difficulties in recruitment, the least dependence on 'helpers', and the majority of student clinical placements. In all ways they were better equipped to provide an occupational therapy service than other areas in the Region. These findings led to close scrutiny of the supply situation to ascertain why this was the case.

The analysis also led to other conclusions being drawn that would be of crucial importance in judging training shortfalls and deciding future policy. Whereas the flows of experienced staff into and out of the Region generally balanced each other out, the Region was a net exporter of newly qualified staff to the extent that twice as many were exported out of the Region as were imported. On examining the operational policies of the training school the reasons for the disparities of employment, and therefore problems in the Region, were clarified. The school took the majority of its intake either from inside its own Area or from outside the Region, and the majority of clinical placements were to be found either in its own Area or outside the Region. As this school was situated in the centre of the Region, both the north and south of the Region were being deprived both of students and clinical placements. An analysis of students' areas of first employment against their area of origin and area of clinical placement during training confirmed that three-quarters of them chose either to return to their home area to work or to the area where they had been placed for clinical training. On average 67 per cent of all students found employment outside the Region, and of those who remained in the Region 84 per cent found employment in the two Authorities closest to the training school. During the four year period studied only three out of the 145 qualifying from the school entered employment in six out of the eight Authorities in the Region.

The synthesis of the demand and supply elements of the report allowed projections of present training policy to be set against the future demands for staff. This enabled a definition of the shortfall of future supply against future demand. In order to overcome such difficulties the Region could adopt one or several policy alternatives. There was the possibility of extension and change of policy at the existing school. But changes in policy on the location of clinical placements and recruitment of students could have an effect on other Regions who at present depended on the Trent school for their qualified staff. Expansion was difficult due to the incapacity of existing facilities to cope with it. Thus a new school was a possibility, perhaps located in the north of the Region to encourage a better level of student recruitment and clinical placements from that area. Other locations for a new school or extensions to other schools outside the Region were studied but the real choice lay in expansion and change of policy at the existing school or the opening of a new school.

The report's main recommendations attempted to sectorise training provision in the Region. It recommended that the present school be retained with its present intake, but that a greater proportion of the intake and clinical placements be obtained from the west and south of the Region. A new school would serve the north and east of the Region, biassing its intakes and clinical placements towards those areas.

Other recommendations (there were 22 in all) suggested policy to help with other specific problems on recruitment, organisation of staff, grading and so on. The final recommendation suggested a policy of continuing to monitor plans, recruitment and wastage rates, training outturns, clinical placements and so on in order to allow policy to be amended quickly and easily as conditions change. The Regional Health Authority accepted the report with a modification that, whilst negotiations should be undertaken with the aim of opening a new school of occupational therapy, the existing school should be expanded in the short term, if at all possible, in order to try to begin to cope with the Region's present and immediate future demands.

The Region has not yet embarked on implementing the policy it has agreed, though it is aware through the comprehensive consultation carried out before it came to its decision that it may encounter difficulties. Though the Region, with the exception of the authority in which the school is situated, is firmly behind the agreed policy, the national bodies controlling training provision are not so convinced. Although they agree the levels of student intake arrived at by the study, their 'territorial policy' on the positioning of training facilities is against any further large expansion nationally (due primarily to shortages of teachers) and would far rather see the expansion being brought about in the present school.

It remains to be seen what the outcome of this particular report on one group of paramedical staff will be, but at least its production has resulted in a Regional policy being agreed and action being planned to overcome present and future staffing problems.

Conclusion

During the conduct of the paramedical studies the manpower planning section in Trent has learned a great deal about the methods, information and 'political' and administrative requirements that suit manpower planning of such staffs in the NHS. It has become obvious that, although the power to alter training policy lies generally at national level, the NHS itself is in a better position to estimate need or demand and can use this knowledge to encourage changes in training policy. An important point in the conduct of manpower planning is where estimates of need are sufficiently local to be realistic and sufficiently central to be able to influence national supply policy. This varies from staff group to staff group in the NHS, and is also influenced by the number and locality of training facilities. In the case of paramedical staff that central point is often at Regional level. In this context the Region is considering defining some training functions, schools and facilities as supra-Area services whose developments will be funded from Region. This will allow flows of staff and Regional needs to be taken into account when the policy of individual training schools is being decided.

The flows of staff, wastage and recruitment rates, return to work rates, outturns of training schools and flows to first employment, and the reasons for these flows, are extremely important factors in planning for professional staff. It is these the manpower planner should seek to influence. In addition a continuous dialogue with the management and the profession concerned in the study plays a vital role not only in ensuring that the best and most comprehensive data is available for analysis, but in order to ensure the commitment of all concerned to the policy arrived at. In many ways planners are, in this context, acting more as recorders of data and opinion, sorters of 'wheat from chaff', and presenters of analyses, rather than being the originators of policy. The continuing dialogues with the profession and management have put manpower planners in Trent in the position of mediators, ensuring that management's requirements are met but also safeguarding the interests of the professions concerned.

The studies have widened manpower planners' knowledge about sources of data. It is often surprising to find what data are available. One such instance involved asking a principal of a training school for information on the area of employment of those qualifying from her school. The researcher was met with blank stares until, on reflection, a book was drawn from a 'dusty drawer', a book in which every student qualifying since the school had opened some years before had been entered, listing their past and present addresses, and past and present posts. This book was kept to invite them to annual reunions at the school.

Finally, such 'one-off' reports as these are valuable in setting a basic direction and acting as a catalyst in the manpower planning. Equally, if not more, important are the resulting monitoring systems necessary, constantly looking at and reassessing the situation as conditions change, and pointing towards desirable amendments to policy in good time to make such changes. Such systems mesh with development of the NHS planning system and by doing so are enhancing the manpower contribution to the system. Thus, through the reports and the monitoring systems that result, manpower planners are beginning to construct the systems the NHS needs in order to adequately plan and utilise its most costly and complex of resources.

NURSING IN THE MENTAL HANDICAP SPECIALTY*

Introduction

The development of a manpower model to investigate the future staffing
levels of nurses of the mentally handicapped arose from a perceived lack
of information available for strategic planning purposes.   The
information routinely available to the Regional Nursing Officer at West
Midlands RHA consisted of numbers of staff in post, for each Area,
District and hospital.   No forecasts of staffing trends or training
requirements were available.   It was therefore essential to find out
current levels of recruitment, training intakes and numbers qualifying,
and to discover the current difficulties and their future implications.
At the same time, concern was expressed about the decline in the size of
nursing intakes into training, due particularly to problems of funding,
(15) and its effect on future (internal) recruitment patterns.

A working party was set up consisting of members of the manpower
planning and operational research sections at the Region, and senior
nurses at Regional, Area and District levels.   Its aim was to
investigate the effects of present and possible future policies of
recruitment and training.   The Regional Nursing Officer wished to know
the training needs for all specialties.   It was decided to tackle one
specialty at a time and mental handicap was chosen because it was self-
contained and the numbers small.   The resultant information would be
used by the Regional care group, assisting in the finalisation of the
strategic plan for the specialty.   Given current thinking on the need
for new community units and the shortage of nurses in the specialty, the
size of training intake to meet such a manpower demand had to be
determined.   A predictive model of recruitment and training levels was
required, in order to assist Areas to predict their own training
requirements.   The same basic model would be used to estimate future
training needs for the other specialties.

Methodology

Four methodological stages were identified, the most critical being the
determination of the manpower structure for nurses of the mentally
handicapped and the identification of flows between grades.   Stage one,
the delineation of the manpower system, was the base upon which the rest
of the work was founded.   It was here that the close involvement with
nursing personnel was essential in order to arrive at a valid manpower
model, and to ensure the full commitment and co-operation of the nursing
staff.   The resultant model of the manpower structure identified the
flows between grades (Figure 3.5, see p.54). (16)

There were two main routes for promotion; one for registered nurses
(RNMS), the other for enrolled nurses (SEN(MS)).   Several subsidiary
paths were also identified.   For learner grades, individuals were

---

*The project reported here was carried out by E.McAleavey (manpower
planning), S.Naylor (operational research), and D.Hassel (Regional
Nurse) for the Regional Nursing Officer at West Midlands RHA in
1977-79.   It has been written up by the editors of this volume;
A.F.Long and G.Mercer.

Fig 3.5 *Model of the Mental Handicap Nursing Structure*

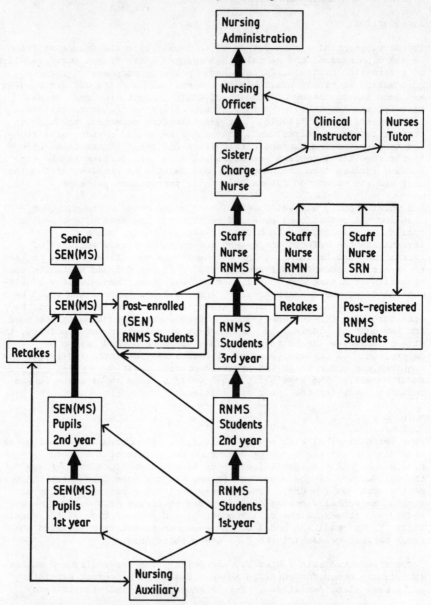

Key: *Only promotion flows are illustrated above. Each grade is also affected by losses due to retirement and wastage, and by gains from external recruitment.*

➤ *indicates the two main promotion routes.*

automatically 'pushed' from one category to another.   Thus in the case
of students a transfer was made to the next year on achieving certain
qualifications or after a prescribed length of service, and to the staff
nurse grade upon successful completion of training.   The alternative to
this Markov assumption was that movement to another category was based
on a renewal process – that is, individuals were 'pulled' in when
vacancies arose.   For example, staff nurses were only promoted to ward
sister level when former members of that grade left or were themselves
promoted.   In fact, staff and enrolled nurses were subject to the
effects of both push and pull mechanisms.

In addition to promotion the system was also affected by losses due to
retirements and wastage, and gains from external recruitment (that is,
recruitment from outside mental handicap nursing, or outside the
Region).   These were all expressed as expected rates per person for
each grade.   In the case of retirement and wastage the rates were
applied to the number of staff in post at the beginning of a year, and
for external recruitment to the number of vacancies arising during that
year.   There were also only two methods of transfer between the
registered and enrolled sections of the structure.   Firstly, RNMS
students might fail their final year examinations but successfully
complete their practical work.   In this case they transferred to
qualified SEN(MS) status.   Similarly, during training, a student might
transfer to pupil training.   Secondly, a qualified SEN(MS) aiming for
higher promotion prospects might achieve registered status by undergoing
a period of post enrolment training.

Having identified a manpower structure and the flow processes, the
second stage in the methodology was to collect the necessary data.   The
model required data on retirement, wastage, and external recruitment
rates for each grade, numbers in post in each grade (in the base year),
and where applicable failure and transfer rates.   From the Regional
payroll information on staff in post in each grade in October 1977 was
obtained.   Numbers of students and pupils, by year of training, were
not easily available from the training schools.   Accordingly, the total
number in training were split to reproduce the effect of current learner
wastage rates.   Information on wastage rates and movements of whole
occupational groups was available, but not for individual grades within
an occupational group.   Figures on retirement and wastage rates for the
last two or three years were obtained from individual hospitals by nurse
members of the working party.   Information patterns of recruitment
relied on the nurses' intuitive estimates, particularly in the case of
external recruitment. (17)

The third stage was to generate forecasts of staff movements on the
basis of current data and estimates of future retirement, wastage and
recruitment patterns.   A manual model and a computer version were
developed.   For the first year of the model the rates of retirement,
wastage and recruitment were applied to current numbers of staff in
each grade.   For subsequent years, the model calculated the expected
numbers in post, and wastage and other rates were applied accordingly.

An illustration of the workings of the model can be seen in Table
3.8 (see p.56) in relation to Figure 3.5.   The study period begins with
30 learners in the second year SEN(MS) category.   All of these were
necessarily pushed into a new 'grade' at the end of the year.   Although

Table 3·8 Estimated Movement between Grades in Mental Handicap Nursing

NUMBER OF STAFF

GRADE	IN POST	RET a	WAST b	CLIN INST c	NURSE TUTOR	POST ENR d	SEN (MS)	RE-TAKE	PROM e	TOTAL LOSS	RNMS	EXT RECR f	INT RECR g	TOTAL INTAKE	NEW NUMBER IN POST REQUIRED
NURSING ADMIN	22	1							2	2		0	2	2	22
NURSING OFFICER	58	0	8						2	10		1	9	10	58
CLINICAL INSTRUCTOR	7	0	0		1				0	1		0	1	1	7
SISTER/CHARGE NURSE	318	22	45	1	0				9	77		0	77	77	318
STAFF NURSE RNMS	116	0	16						77	93		0/P	73/96	93/P	119
STAFF NURSE RMN, SRN	30	0	5			5				10		10		10	30
REG REG RNMS STUDENTS	5		0						5	5			5	5	5
POST ENR SEN STUDENTS	16		0						16	16			16	16	16
STUDENT RETAKES	8		2				0	0	6	8			7	7	7
RNMS STUDENTS 3rd YEAR	80		2				2	7	69	80			74	74	74
RNMS STUDENTS 2nd YEAR	85		11				0		74	85			83	83	83
RNMS STUDENTS 1st YEAR	93		10				0		83	93		84	9	93	93
NURSING AUXILIARIES	911	5	19						9	33		33		33	911
SENIOR SEN (MS)	41	0	0							0	0	0	0	0	41
SEN (MS)	360	14	50			16			0	80	2	0/P	78/32	80/P	314
PUPIL RETAKES	10		0					4	10	10		4		4	4
SEN (MS) PUPILS 2nd YEAR	30		4						22	30	0		35	35	35
SEN (MS) PUPILS 1st YEAR	53		18						35	53		26	27	53	53
NURSING AUXILIARIES	911								27	27		27	0	27	911

KEY: a, Retirement; b, Wastage; c, Clinical Instructor; d, Post Enrolled; e, Promotion; f, External Recruitment; g, Internal Recruitment

there were 30 losses, there were only 22 of this group promoted to the
staff nurse grade since four had left entirely, and another four had to
retake their exams.   The overall gains to the enrolled nurse category
however amounted to 32 persons, since there were 10 others who has
successfully retaken their second year exams.   Despite these gains and
the transfer of two nurses from the RNMS path, the overall wastage
reduced the SEN strength from 360 to 314 at the end of the year.   That
diminution might be counterbalanced by external recruitment, but this
lay outside the scope of the model.

The computer model produced the results of these calculations at
yearly intervals for the next 10 years.   A percentage split between
trained staff, learners and untrained staff, and between registered and
enrolled staff, was also produced for each year, so that the likely
future balance between different groups of staff could be monitored.
Such results were then available to the care group considering the
future of the Region's services for the mentally handicapped.

The final stage in the study was to examine the sensitivity of the
model and its output and thus its fit to real life career structures.
The model's sensitivity to changes in wastage and retirement rates was
explored.   In general, the model highlighted the fact that the
fluctuation in the wastage and retirement rates of staff nurse or SEN
grades will have a disproportionate effect on other grades.   The larger
the number of people in post in a grade, the greater will be the effect
of any change.   This in turn would affect the shortage or surplus of
qualifying students and may change third year student wastage and
external recruitment to staff nurses, if more or fewer qualifiers were
to be appointed.

It was a characteristic of the manpower model that changes occurring
in the promotion routes for registered or enrolled nurses always
affected the balance between qualifiers and number of vacancies at staff
nurse or SEN level.   This occurred even when numbers in post at other
grades were unaffected.   Considerable emphasis had therefore to be
placed on the supply and demand for nurses at these levels.   An
examination of external recruitment, at present excluded from the model,
would improve its fit to the real life situation.   This will come about
as a result of the development of a nursing manpower data base set up in
the Region.

The critical points in the methodology are summarised in Table 3.9
(see p.58).   It was essential to arrive at an appropriate and realistic
model of the manpower system and to identify the flows between grades.
The commitment of the nursing staff to the model representing the
manpower structure and their involvement in producing the model were
indispensable to the progress of the study.

Table 3.9
Summary of the Methodological Approach

Stage One   Delineate the manpower structure.   Identify the
               flows into, out of, and between grades (recruit-
               ment, promotion, retirement, wastage).   Identify
               the push/pull process.

Stage Two   Identify and collect necessary data (retirement,
               wastage, recruitment, staff in post - preferably
               by age, sex, grade, qualification, and hospital).

Stage Three Generate the forecasts required on the basis of
               alternative assumptions.   Examine the implications
               for training intake numbers and external/internal
               recruitment.

Stage Four   Examine the sensitivity of the model to changes in
               wastage, retirement rates and external recruitment.

Discussion

This simulation model has been used to demonstrate the effects of
inequalities at the point where the push/pull mechanisms meet (at the
grades of staff nurse, (RNMS) or SEN(MS)), and to suggest possible
outcomes.   For example, if the model suggested that the demand for
staff nurses will be greater than the supply from the student grades,
then one possibility would be to attempt to increase external recruitment.   Another approach would be to increase student intakes and/or
attempt to reduce wastage at the student and registered nurse level.
If both these policies failed the result would be a reduction in staff
in post with a consequent effect on patient care.   The efficiency of
such decisions can be assessed in the model, through altering recruitment levels and wastage rates appropriately.   In other words, the focus
and emphasis of the model and its output is not to provide a definitive
view of the future, but to enable comparisons to be made of the effects
of different policies.

The forecasts of manpower needs for nurses in the mental handicap
specialty presented in the Regional strategy highlight the use made of
the model for strategic planning.   The resultant manpower forecasts
have clear implications for training intake levels at the Area level.
As was stated in the Regional plan, 'long-term staffing difficulties can
be overcome provided authorities develop training strategies now and
monitor their progress.' (18)   In consultation with the Areas, the
Region will have to explore how they will meet this training need.   The
concern is not only how to increase training intakes, but also how to
reduce wastage within training.   Independently of the model, Directors
of Nurse Education will have to concentrate attention on how wastage can
be reduced, by reviewing selection procedures or by focusing on the
numbers and use of tutorial staff.

The model was concerned primarily with the supply of nurses, assuming
that the current staffing levels were to be maintained.   The facilities
exist to increase (or decrease) these levels by a given proportion in
any one year.   There is a need, however, to define future staffing

levels (manpower demand) to take account of such things as split wards, limited suitable clinical experiences, increased numbers of community staff, a shorter working week for nurses, the potential implications of the Jay Report, (19) and the expected rundown of hospital beds in the specialty in the Region, so that more realistic establishment assumptions can be used. It would also be of value to apply the model to funded establishments for the determination of vacancies, as well as the present focus on staff in post.

The model has, therefore, the necessary flexibility to explore various assumptions about the future and possible policies. Its aid to strategic planning as a tool indicating the outcomes of alternative policies is clear. The potential exists for the model, suitably altered, to be extended to apply to other nursing divisions and other staff groups - that is, to any group which has a graded structure.

However, the project was not without its drawbacks. Problems arose in the area of data, once the manpower structure and flows were identified. The data on wastage, retirement and recruitment were not readily available for each grade. In fact, the data used for external recruitment were estimated by the nursing personnel. Age specific data would enable more sophisticated manpower planning models, such as those available in the set of Civil Service models known as MANPLAN, to be assessed for their applicability to nursing manpower structures. (20) To this end, work has been set under way to generate information demanded by such models.

Conclusion

The value of this case study can be briefly summarised. Firstly, the project was based on a fairly straightforward and simple approach to the problem exploring the effect on staffing levels of the movement of nursing staff in mental handicap within the West Midlands RHA. The project, a joint one between members of the operational research and manpower planning sections in conjunction with nursing personnel, involved a learning process for all concerned. In particular the nursing staff became aware of the need to explore and take into account levels of wastage, retirement, and so on when making decisions about training intakes. Goodwill and commitment existed in the Region to this exercise and its conclusions.

Secondly, the critical aspect of the whole project was the development of the model, the identification of the flows, and the push/pull mechanisms. Without a good and realistic model, little progress would have been made. The importance of joint working with the nurses was apparent. Such a joint approach is very different to one of going out to Areas, telling them that this is the model, and that these are the data requirements.

The concern for simplicity inevitably meant that certain aspects of the situation were explored only marginally or not at all. For example, although mention was made of external recruitment (recruitment of qualified staff from outside of the output of the training school), no attempt was made to assess the feasibility of this option. No labour market analysis was carried out, although the Regional Nursing Department was examining the capacity of the training schools to increase intakes and liaising with the Regional Nurse Training Council regarding future needs for tutorial staff. The same comment applies to increases in training intake. In addition, use was made of limited data, even intuitive guesses, as inputs to the model. An accurate data base for nursing manpower is currently being developed which will enable the model to be rerun accordingly. The intention was to return to these issues and explore their implications once the model was accepted as being a valuable aid to strategic planning.

The modelling work described in this paper has its limitations. The choice of the mental handicap specialty was deliberate. Whilst the methodology can be straightforwardly applied and generalised to other nursing divisions and occupational groups, its complexity increases. For example, looking at the general nursing division, a nurse who leaves the hospital and moves to another hospital in the same Area can be viewed as wastage (to the hospital of origin) or as internal movement (at an Area level). Again a movement from one Area to another is wastage at this level and at the Regional level internal movement. Accordingly, the manpower system and possible flows become more complex and numerous. The model is thus best operated at a District or even Area level and not on an individual hospital basis. Indeed, a strong case could be put for disaggregating the analysis and carrying out the calculations of the model for each health authority involved, and aggregating at the end to arrive at the Regional picture.

The final comment relates to the output of the model. It only provides a range of future possible outcomes on the basis of alternative assumptions and policies. It does not and cannot generate answers. It is a practical aid to decision making, examining alternative policies for strategic planning.

NOTES

(1)   DHSS, Medical Manpower - The Next Twenty Years, HMSO, London 1978.
(2)   G.McLachlan, B.Stocking and R.F.A.Shegog (eds), Patterns for
Uncertainty? Planning for the Greater Medical Profession, Nuffield
Provincial Hospitals Trust, Oxford University Press, Oxford 1979.
(3)   DHSS, Medical Manpower, Ch.IV, 'Demand'.
(4)   Ibid., p.14 and p.20.
(5)   Ibid., p.21.
(6)   Wessex Regional Health Authority, Wessex Regional Plan, Paper
R529, 1979.
(7)   Trent's occupational therapists grew by 115 per cent during the 10
years studied.
(8)   Whereas Trent had 3.5 occupational therapists per 100,000
population in 1976, and the national average was 4.6 per 100,000
population, in 1988 the national average was assessed to be 6.3 per
100,000 population.
(9)   The present best staffed Region - Oxford - had 6.8 occupational
therapists per 100,000 population in 1976. It is interesting to note
that if Trent was able to staff up to its establishment levels it would
have had 6.2 staff per 100,000 population in 1978, very near to the
suggested national average level for 1988.
(10) The analysis of projected 'national averages' and 'best Region'
levels can be criticised as chasing the staffing levels of other Regions
and not being a true estimation of need. The analysis of capital
developments can be criticised as being based on the old adage of 'think
of a number and double it'. The estimate from strategic plans,
although perhaps having most intrinsic validity, was based on only a
25 per cent sample of all Areas and as later analysis showed was awry by
some 16 per cent. The analysis of past spending patterns had the
advantage of restraining staffing levels within likely financial
availability, but again, as later analysis of plans showed, the way in
which Authorities spent their revenue in the past is not necessarily a
good method of assessing how they will spend it in the future, and
indeed is based on a level of expenditure which is itself constrained by
a lack of availability of occupational therapists to employ. The
levels of increase suggested by the analyses were as follows: projected
'national average' level, 83 per cent; projected 'best Region' level,
145 per cent; capital developments, 163 per cent; estimate from
strategic plans, 108 per cent; and previous spending patterns, 73 per
cent.
(11) In the last 10 years the actual increase in numbers had been 99
compared with the future decade projection of a further 180 staff.
Then again, in 1978 Trent was 106 occupational therapists short of its
'funded' establishment levels.
(12) This amounted to 20 posts.
(13) The origin of applicants was in the ratio of one from the area of
the training school to three from the rest of the Region to 20 from
outside the Region. The origin of students was in the ratio of one
from the area of the training school to 1.5 from the Region to 9.5 from
outside the Region.
(14) The alternatives were: to expand at the present school; to move
the school elsewhere in the centre of the Region; to provide an
additional school in the centre of the Region; to move the school to
the north of the Region; to provide an additional school in the north
of the Region; and to encourage expansion in other schools outside the

Region.

(15) Birmingham AHA(T) in particular was experiencing problems due to a decline in revenue (through Regional RAWP). It also expressed the view that it was training not only for itself, but for the whole Region and thus more money should be forthcoming.

(16) A similar approach, developing a model of the manpower structure, was involved in a South East Thames RHA project. See Regional Nursing and Midwifery Committee, Manpower Planning for Nursing and Midwifery Staff, South East Thames Regional Health Authority, March 1979.

(17) It was intended that the model could run on a Regional average set of figures. However, considerable variation between hospitals was apparent. Accordingly, the model was examined using data for one hospital and the effects of changes in the data were explored.

(18) West Midlands Regional Health Authority, Regional Strategy 1979-1988, vol.3, 1979, p.20.

(19) Committee of Enquiry into Mental Handicapped Nursing and Care, Report, (Jay Report), Cmnd. 7468, HMSO, London 1979. Estimates of the future demand were made by the care group examining staffing for the new County Units.

(20) Tentative use was made of one such model - the KENT model. This is a general forecasting model, requiring age specific input data. It was used to explore the structure of mental handicap nursing in relation to its promotion aspects. See Civil Service Department, A Management Guide to Manpower Planning Models, HMSO, London 1975, Chapter 8. One problem would however be a possible loss in understanding by the nurses involved in the project, and a potential shift in emphasis to system modelling.

4 A Manpower Information System
J. Cree

'The development of manpower planning in the NHS has been
hampered - if not entirely prevented - by the lack of accurate
information about the staff employed . . . This situation should
be rectified by the provision of the Standard Manpower Planning
and Personnel Information System (STAMP).'

Many managers in the NHS have, at some time over the last few years,
heard or read such a statement.   To some it may have acted as a
reassurance that the problems they were facing in trying to do some
manpower planning were common to all and that a solution to these
problems was imminent.   This chapter attempts to put STAMP into context
and to show that as a standardised, national system it can only act as
the foundation for the subsequent development of comprehensive manpower
information systems in the NHS.   It will also become clear that rather
than being a solution to manpower planning difficulties, STAMP may
create new and additional problems because the NHS will have to learn
how to use the information provided.   Indeed, the historical lack of
relevant information about manpower could be attributable to a general
failure to tackle manpower problems.

The chapter begins with a brief overview of the state of manpower
information in the NHS and a description of the background against
which the need for a standardised system was first identified.   It
then turns to the way in which the development of STAMP was undertaken
and highlights the reasons behind the adopted approach together with
some of the problems encountered along the way.   A description of the
system, the information held and the ways in which the information can
be made available to users is also given.   The chapter concludes with
some examples of how manpower information can be used in the planning
and control of NHS manpower and shows how far STAMP is able to provide
the necessary details.

BACKGROUND TO MANPOWER INFORMATION IN THE NHS

Each year the DHSS requires health authorities to provide a census of
all employees. (1)   In the past the information has been submitted by
the manual completion of forms listing numbers and whole-time

equivalents of each type of staff employed at a particular point each year. These forms were completed by every authority and proved to be a time consuming task. The results were regarded by authorities as a prime source of manpower information; partly because locally produced information was generally regarded as more dependable than that output from a Regional Computer Centre, and partly because other sources of manpower information may not have been available. The difficulties with these annual censuses were that they only related to one point in a year and, as the year progressed, the data became increasingly obsolete. In addition, despite considerable efforts nationally and locally, many errors and omissions occurred. Often those completing the forms, which were lengthy and fairly detailed, were not those who were going to use that information. Also, in places where there were alternative sources of manpower data, the completion of the census forms was regarded as just another 'DHSS requirement'. Priority was not always given to ensuring that all of the data were accurate.

The introduction of the Standard Payroll System (SPS) in the NHS allows for the automatic submission of census information from computer files. (2) This facility is available to all Regions using SPS and, in addition, to those who can add to their local pay schemes the data items required for the census. It should remove many of the inaccuracy problems of manual returns and allow useful comparisons of staffing levels between Regions. But it still provides no more than an annual stocktaking of numbers employed and, as such, has a limited role to play in the field of manpower information needs.

The prime source of regular information about NHS employees has been the data held on Regional computers for pay purposes. Most Regions had their own systems to extract certain personal details on employees from each month's payroll and to provide standard outputs or schedules of this information. Typically, the outputs consisted of nominal rolls giving individual information; head counts giving summarised statistics on numbers employed by different grades, locations and sex; crude turnover and stability indices for different staff groups at different locations; and retirement schedules.

Such schedules have been, and in many places still are, the only regular source of information about all employees and have been used by a variety of managers - personnel officers, manpower planners, nursing officers and accountants. For example, nominal rolls provided personnel officers with the equivalent of an employee index whilst accountants used them in the process of setting up budgets. The statistical head counts were used to monitor changes in staffing levels and assisted in the completion of various DHSS statistical returns. Occasionally, the dates of birth found on the nominal rolls were used for analyses of age structures whilst the turnover data might be studied for indications of excessive wastage levels. The schedule provided a considerable amount of basic data on every employee but the information tended to be used mainly as reference material in case of enquiry. Very seldom was the data manipulated or analysed in a way useful for manpower planning purposes.

A major reason for the failure to exploit this information was that the standard schedules provided to users rarely satisfied all their requirements. What they needed might well have been contained somewhere in the schedules but it often required considered manual effort to extract and analyse it in a way suitable for their purpose. Only the most dogged user will persist in the task of searching through large piles of computer printout to uncover the particular items required before analysis can begin. A second reason that this information was not fully utilised lay in the drawbacks inherent in relying upon payroll as the source of manpower data. In many cases the ways in which a payroll classifies staff are not appropriate for personnel or manpower planning purposes. For example, the NHS planning system demands a care group classification of staff but the payroll system does not provide this facility. The same problem occurs in relation to the classification of work, such as nursing divisions or specialties. Another complication is that some of the data held on the payroll system which are used for manpower purposes are not essential for pay purposes. Prime examples of this are items such as date of birth and date of joining the authority. Neither of these. are accorded a high priority when it comes to ensuring accuracy of payroll records.

To reject the payroll as a source of manpower data would, however, be foolish. Much of the information held on payroll records is necessary for manpower planning and personnel work. To set up a separate system which duplicated payroll data would be extravagant and would inevitably lead to inconsistencies between the two systems. Many of the payroll 'anomalies' could be removed if users of manpower information took the trouble to work more closely with their financial colleagues. Even for those anomalies that persist, an understanding of the effect they have on the manpower data would provide users with greater confidence in the data.

The inadequacy of payroll derived manpower data has been felt most strongly by local managers who required information which was not available from the routine schedules or who found that the manual effort required to extract the relevant data from those schedules too time consuming. Departmental managers have needed to keep their own manual records on staff sickness, holidays, staff changes, overtime, shift rotas, and so on, for use in controlling their establishment.

These manual systems vary in the amount of information they hold but even an employee's original application form will provide many pieces of information such as previous career history and qualifications which are not to be found on any payroll record. In general, however, such information is never summarised or analysed on a regular basis. The problem with all manual information systems is that once the amount of data held exceeds that level at which regular manual analysis is easy or even possible they lose much of their usefulness. Very little attention has been paid to the possibility of capturing these data and summarising them for use at authority level whilst still allowing the local manager to make use of the initial input documents in the day to day running of the department.

There are a number of other local manpower information systems which have been developed within the NHS in attempts to overcome the deficiencies of the purely payroll based or purely manual systems. Firstly, Cambridge District, within the East Anglian Regional Health Authority, has developed a personnel information system which combines many of the advantages of payroll extracted and manually based

methods. (3)   In addition to the routine schedules produced from
payroll a considerable amount of additional data is collected on
standard forms at the time of appointment or departure of individual
members of staff and stored in the computer.   The difficulty that this
system confronts is that whilst many other authorities have expressed an
interest in the outputs they are doubtful whether the benefits of such a
system justify the time or expense required to add the non payroll data
to the system.   This problem faces anyone attempting to market a
manpower information system which requires user effort.   Although there
are many cries for more manpower information in the NHS, few people know
what they would use the information for and do not consider the
collection of manpower data to have a very high priority.

Secondly, there have been several small systems developed by different
authorities which deal with the recording and analysis of a few non
payroll items of information such as qualifications and absence.   The
problem here lies in the fact that one major benefit of having such
information held on the computer should be the ability to combine it
with other computerised personal information extracted from payroll or
from other sources.   For example, if information on the type and
duration of absences from work could be combined with information on
overtime hours worked or the use of agency and other temporary labour
together with the associated costs, it is possible to derive not only an
analysis of how many hours had been lost to the service but also the
manpower and financial consequences of making good this lost time.   The
reasons for this lack of integration are mainly concerned with the
difficulties of linking with payroll systems, particularly with SPS.
In addition, few people have attempted to draw up an overall framework
for their manpower information requirements, with the result that a
rather inefficient, piecemeal approach to the problem has grown, like
Topsy, as each new problem arose.

To sum up, purely manual manpower information systems are untenable
in the NHS, considering the number of employees.   Those who could
obtain information from their payroll system were suspicious of its
authenticity or deemed it inappropriate for the purposes they had in
mind.   Others were not even making use of the payroll data they
received because they perceived no need to do so.   Those who claimed
they required more information than payroll provided faced the problem
of gaining the commitment and resources necessary to obtain it.   There
were also the difficulties of reaching agreement with other users on
what information should be collected and how it should be analysed and
output.   Where these hurdles were overcome there was the danger of
developing a variety of manpower systems, none of which linked with or
enhanced the benefits of the others.

The increasing variety of approaches adopted to provide manpower
information and the varying degrees of interest and expertise in its use
were making it extremely difficult to obtain comparable data on the NHS
as a whole.   In addition, it was desirable to avoid duplication of
effort across the country as each authority attempted to provide its own
solution to the growing demand.   It was against this background that
STAMP was generated to provide a national solution.

DEVELOPMENT AND APPROACH OF STAMP

In 1971 the Secretary of State for Health and Social Services announced
that there was to be a policy of standardisation for NHS computing.
This was an attempt to achieve compatability of equipment and systems
throughout the NHS and to prevent overlap in development effort.   It
was not until 1975 that a manpower and personnel information system was
proposed as the basis for a standard NHS package.   Perhaps the major
incentives behind this proposal were the inability of the DHSS to obtain
accurate and consistent data on the staff employed in the NHS, the fact
that reorganisation had created formal personnel and manpower planning
functions, and the subsequent formation of MAPLIN which initially was a
forum for discussions on the need for more and better manpower
information. (4)

  Responsibility for the development of a standard manpower planning and
personnel information system was allocated to Wessex in late 1975.
From the start it was assumed by the National Standardisation Committee
that this manpower system would be firmly linked to payroll to avoid
unnecessary duplication of information collection.   Moreover, the
payroll system referred to was SPS whose development was already well
under way within the North Western Region.   Almost as soon as work on
the development of STAMP commenced it was found that it would have to be
in two stages; interim and main STAMP.   SPS was already being adopted
by some Regions and where these had been using manpower systems linked
to their own local payroll they were being left without any regular
manpower data.   It was therefore agreed that the first task for Wessex
had to be the rapid development of a manpower system which would operate
against SPS.   Such a system would be a temporary measure until the
STAMP system proper was available.   Wessex commenced work immediately
and due to the urgency of the system proceeded with minimal consultation
on the design, basing its ideas on the sort of system it had been
operating for the last few years.   This temporary system became known
as interim STAMP.

  Interim STAMP as first released brought into full view several
important problems.   The complexity of SPS had been severely under-
estimated and too little effort had been put into that part of the
interim system which operated against SPS.   This difficulty was
exacerbated because Wessex itself was not using SPS.   Testing of the
interim system was only possible after its release to other user
Regions.   Interim STAMP underwent continual revision and enhancement
until a final version was produced for release in 1978.   It was
entirely parasitic upon SPS in that all its data were taken from SPS.
There was no facility to add non payroll data.   In addition, the data
extracted from SPS concerned personal details only; no financial
information was captured by interim STAMP.   Outputs from the interim
system consisted of an age analysis, a nominal roll, an hours analysis,
head counts by financial code and by authority, a retirement schedule,
and a starters and leavers analysis.

  Interim STAMP was used by six Regions: Oxford; Northern; South
West Thames; North East Thames; East Anglia; and Wessex.   The
remaining Regions were either not using SPS or, as in the case of Mersey
and North Western, had developed their own manpower systems to operate
against SPS.   In its final version, interim STAMP met with considerable

approval, and represented a substantial advance upon previously operated local systems. However, while the standard schedules were initially welcomed by the Regions, as the users gained experience and expertise in handling the data, requests for changes and additions to the outputs flowed into Wessex. Alterations to the layout, to the totalling facilities, and to the content of the outputs were the most frequent suggestions for amendment but these requests obviously varied according to the specific needs of each user.

Both the time it took to devise the interim system and the feedback received from users were valuable in assisting the development of main STAMP. Firstly, a thorough knowledge of SPS had been gained. Secondly, it was obvious that many managers in the NHS were only just beginning to understand the uses and benefits of manpower information. They needed time to absorb the interim system before even more information was handed out. Thirdly, the differing output requirements and the difficulty in getting users to agree on a format have brought home the practical problems in catering for a wide range of user needs. All too often problems and tasks have not been thought through to a precise definition of the sort of analysis required. Finally, the term 'user' extended more widely than originally envisaged. Interest in STAMP and feedback on the interim system has come from managers at all levels and from many different functions. It became obvious that STAMP was going to cater for more than just the manpower planning and personnel specialists.

The design of the main STAMP system was based on a number of criteria. It had to be simple enough in its basic form for all users to understand. It had to be sufficiently flexible to allow users to specify the levels of aggregation, the types of analysis, and the design of the outputs to satisfy their own particular requirements. The system also had to be modular and mainly optional so that users could implement parts of the system as and when the desire and capacity arose. Finally, the system had to be cheap to operate.

With these criteria in mind it was decided that main STAMP should consist of a core of SPS derived data to which additional information, not available from SPS, could be added if and when a user authority wished to do so. The SPS data include all items previously captured by the interim system but in addition main STAMP extracts all of the financial data on each employee considered useful for manpower purposes. This part of the system that extracted SPS data and set up basic STAMP records for each individual is labelled module one and is the sole compulsory module of main STAMP. As part of this first module all the standard schedules (with some of the amendments suggested by users of the interim system) previously produced from interim STAMP are available, together with two additional standard outputs: a master file print and a cost analysis print. The master file print shows all the data held on an individual by the STAMP computer record. This enables each member of staff to check on the information held and its accuracy. A sample of the printout can be seen in Appendix 1. The cost analysis print provides a breakdown of staff costs incurred week by week, within each cost centre and expense number as identified on the Standard Accounting System (SAS). (5) Only those Regions using SPS, SAS, and STAMP can obtain the cost analysis printout. Table 4.1 provides a summary of the contents of each of the standard schedules available with main STAMP. (6)   The second module of main STAMP comprises the facility by which users can add items of information, not available from SPS, onto an employee's individual record (the basis of module one). Currently, Wessex have allowed for the input of date of start in the NHS, nationality, and ethnic origin.

Table 4.1
Standard Printouts Available in Main STAMP

Nominal Roll	A list of staff employed on a particular date, giving location, name, age, sex, marital status, grade, occupation, date appointed, and whole-time equivalent.
Headcount by Financial Code	Numbers (and wte) of staff employed on a particular date, subdivided by location of work, payscale, occupation, and sex.
Headcount by NHS Authority	Numbers (and wte) of staff employed on a particular date, subdivided by payscale and occupation within an entire NHS authority.
Starters and Leavers Analysis	Numbers (and wte) of starters and leavers in a specified period, sub-divided by employing authority, occupation, grade, and sex, giving turnover and stability indices and reasons for leaving.
Hours Analysis	A monthly breakdown of hours worked by each employee, showing hours worked at basic, enhanced, and overtime rates.
Retirement Schedule	A nominal roll of staff due to retire in the following five years, giving name, location, grade, occupation, sex, age, and date of retirement.
Age Analysis	Number of staff in post on a particular date, subdivided by grade, occupation, sex, and age.
Master File Print	A printout of each employee's main STAMP record, showing all the information held on STAMP about that employee.
Cost Analysis Print	A breakdown of the staff costs incurred week by week, by type of cost, and by each SAS expense number within a particular cost centre.

The first two modules of STAMP were made available to the NHS in July 1980, together with the standard schedules.   The third module, to be available in January 1981 in time to allow the collection and input of data for the September submission of medical and dental returns, is a system whereby the various statutory returns to the DHSS on medical staff employed can be provided on computer tape. As much of the information required by the DHSS (and currently submitted manually) is not available on SPS, the medical statistics module will necessitate the direct input of additional data to STAMP. Regions which take up this module will be able to dispense with the manual completion of all medical and dental returns and will also gain a complete and accurate in post record for use in medical staff planning.

Further information can be added to main STAMP through the development of another module. Suggested modules include ones on qualifications, absence, and establishment control. Each will require the collection and direct input of information not held on SPS. Any NHS authority can develop its own module or make use of one already developed by another authority. Wessex will only be responsible for linking additional modules to module one of main STAMP. One important requirement in the development of further modules is that classifications adopted are standard throughout the NHS. For example, a user wishing to collect and input qualifications data would have to base the input upon an agreed list of qualifications. Responsibility for devising such standard classifications rests upon the NHS and DHSS officers represented on MAPLIN. (7)

In addition to the standard schedules, Wessex is providing a simple computer enquiry system called Design-A-Form which allows users with no knowledge of computer programming to obtain printouts of STAMP information tailormade to their own needs. There are two parts to Design-A-Form: a print programme library and user designed prints. The print programme library is a collection of programmes which have already been written by various Regions to analyse STAMP information. The format of the library prints is fixed, but users can specify which staff group they want analysed. All a user has to do to obtain a library print is to specify the reference number of the particular programme and the staff group required. The prints available in the library will increase steadily as Regions add new programmes. An example of one print available in the library is shown in Appendix 2. The second part of Design-A-Form is the facility for users to design their own nominal roll and head count printouts. (8) In addition to Design-A-Form, considerable efforts have been made to make the STAMP data easily accessible to ad hoc investigation, using the enquiry packages available with ICL computers, such as FILETAB. These will be added to the Design-A-Form library. The ad hoc enquiry approach to obtaining manpower information thus offers individually styled reports which should largely obviate the need for manual analyses.

The development of both the interim and main STAMP systems has proved to be much more difficult and time consuming than was envisaged. Many of the problems experienced in relation to the interim system stemmed from a gross underestimation of the complexity of SPS. However, not all of the difficulties have emanated from Wessex or STAMP. Firstly, STAMP relies heavily on SPS, and as a standard system, must assume that SPS is used in every Region in the ways intended by its North Western sponsor. Inevitably, payroll departments in some Regions have introduced their own 'short cuts' which can adversely affect the manpower data derived from STAMP. Secondly, it must be remembered that the computer only operates on the information it receives. The adage 'rubbish in - rubbish out' is often forgotten and STAMP has been blamed for inaccuracies which it is the responsibility of the user to correct. Finally, the requirements of users change very rapidly as experience of manpower information is accumulated, and it is most difficult to design a system that will keep up with these constantly changing demands. Design-A-Form, however, should go a long way towards providing the flexibility users require.

STAMP has often been viewed with suspicion. As the best advertisement for any product is an example of its applicability, the successful implementation and operation of the interim system has gone some way to engender confidence in prospective users. This increased confidence, together with the availability of financial information on main STAMP, and the Design-A-Form facility is beginning to engender a much more positive approach to STAMP in the NHS. Currently, it is expected that 10 of the 14 English health Regions will be using the main STAMP system by April 1981.

USES OF MANPOWER INFORMATION

Up to now this chapter has discussed the provision of manpower information with little mention of how this might be utilised. This section outlines three areas where manpower information has a contribution to make and shows how far STAMP, in terms of its payroll derived data, can provide assistance.

Staffing a new unit

There have been numerous occasions where a new development has not been able to open as planned due to the inability to provide the necessary staff to run it. In this example the steps that could be taken to avoid that eventuality are examined. Ideally, of course, there should be an investigation into the staffing consequences before any new development is actually carried out. In this way it should be possible to influence the siting, the size, or the facilities to be provided in order to maximise the chances of attracting the necessary staff. This has rarely happened in the past. It is more often the case that those responsible for staffing are presented with a final development plan and simply asked to ensure that the staff are there when they are needed. Whichever the case the sort of questions to be asked about manpower are similar.

The example is concerned with the development of a new 50 bed unit on the site of the existing District General Hospital (DGH). The unit is due for completion in eight years' time. The District Nursing Officer (DNO), who has been having some problems in finding the nurses to staff existing services, is worried about how to find additional personnel.

The first step is to assess the size of the problem. As the new unit will only be one part of the staffing requirements in eight years' time the number required for the whole of the DGH site must be calculated. To make the exercise manageable the nursing workforce is initially divided into qualified and unqualified staff categories. Once likely problems have been identified, the staffing situation can be examined in

more detail.   The head count information received from STAMP indicates
that the average number of nurses employed at the DGH is 375 whole-time
equivalents (wte), of which 60 per cent are qualified and 40 per cent
unqualified.   In addition, it is known through STAMP that there is a
total of 125 student and pupil nurses at various stages of their
training.   Excluding the learners the nursing staff are servicing 510
beds which means that the current nursing ratio is 0.73 wte nurses per
bed.   The DGH is currently short of nurses, and a further 23 nurses are
needed to bring the workforce up to strength, leading to a nursing ratio
of 0.78 wte nurses per bed.   To staff the total of 560 beds at the
opening of the new unit it is therefore estimated that 437 wte are
required.   If the current proportions of qualified to unqualified staff
are maintained, an additional 37 wte qualified nurses and 25 wte
unqualified nurses must be recruited.   The details are summarised in
Table 4.2.

Table 4.2
Nursing Staff Requirements

Current Position

Average number of nurses employed at the DGH	375 wte	to 510 beds
Qualified (60%)	225	
Unqualified (40%)	150	
Total number of student and pupil nurses in training	125	
Current ratio of nurses to beds (excluding students and pupils)	0.73	
Current staffing norm, nurses to beds (excluding students and pupils)	0.78	
Current staffing requirement (shortfall)	23 wte	

Future Position

To staff the DGH and the new unit on the basis of the current staffing norm (0.78 nurses to a bed)	437 wte	to 560 beds
To maintain 60:40 split of qualified to unqualified staff		
Additional qualified staff required	37 wte	
Additional unqualified staff required	25 wte	
Total additional staff required		
To staff 560 beds on the basis of 0.78 nurses to a bed	62 wte	
To maintain existing workforce to replace losses due to turnover	110 wte per annum	

These additions seemed relatively small and the DNO, at first glance,
could see no real problems in finding the extra staff.   On further
reflection it was recognised that some of the existing staff would
leave in the next eight years, whether because of retirement or some
other reason.   The STAMP retirement schedule indicated that a total of
35 nurses were due for retirement over the next five years.   The STAMP
age analysis showed that a further 40 were aged between 50 and 55 years
and were also likely to retire just before, or soon after, the new unit
opened.   A glance at the turnover figures for nurses at the DGH over

the last year indicated that 25 per cent of the qualified nurses and 32 per cent of the unqualified nurses had left. When the consequences of leavers had been calculated, it was found that instead of just 62 extra staff to be recruited for the new unit, in each of the next 8 years approximately 110 additional nurses would also have to be found, assuming constant turnover rates. At this stage the calculations were becoming rather complicated and the DNO suspected that they were too crude to represent an accurate picture of staffing flows, and asked for technical assistance.

There are various computer techniques available which can model a situation such as the one confronting the DNO and can carry out the rather tedious and time consuming calculations necessary to forecast, over a period of time, the likely flows of manpower and the implications of these on the staff available. (9)   These models vary in their level of sophistication.   The required data could be taken directly from STAMP.   The basic information would consist of the wte unqualified and qualified nurses in post at the time at the DGH, categorised by their age and length of service, together with the average turnover rates associated with each age/length of service group over the last few years.

The first run of the model would show the DNO what the staffing picture would be each year over the next eight years if there was no recruitment.   From this baseline various actions could be tested for their influence on staffing levels.   From the STAMP records the numbers and characteristics of the staff acquired in the past could be identified.   The implications of maintaining previous policies could be tested.   The effect of increasing recruitment levels could also be explored.   The records held at the local school of nursing would indicate how many of the original intake took up post at the DGH, thus allowing the investigation of the effects of increasing the number of newly qualified recruits.   If the numbers the model estimated would be available were still insufficient, ways of reducing the wastage levels could be explored through such measures as the provision of a creche or additional residential accommodation.   Further possibilities would be to examine the effects of altering the proportion of qualified to unqualified nurses or the results of recruiting already trained nurses from a higher age bracket than was usual from the school of nursing. In addition the increases in staffing would have to be timed so that the required levels were available for the eighth year.   Accordingly, the annual costs involved in carrying an excess of nurses until the new unit opened would need to be weighed.   Throughout this process the DNO would have to confront a range of factors which affect wastage, and understand what might be achieved and what policies would have to be adopted to ensure that nursing levels were satisfactory.   Progress over the next eight years would have to be monitored and, if necessary, the consequences of alternative corrective actions explored.

From this brief description it can be seen how STAMP could provide the framework for the investigation of the problem.   Most of the basic data could be derived from STAMP, whilst the model simply lifts the analytical burden off the user.   Equally essential to the process, however, is the DNO's own awareness of possible problems, the ability to structure an approach to their investigation, indicating what questions to ask, and how to use the available manpower information.

It is also necessary to translate the knowledge of the District - the local labour market, the past recruitment problems, the school of nursing's capacity and the staffing requirements of the DGH - into practical courses of action. This information is equally as important as the hard data available from such a system as STAMP for nurse manpower planning.

Budgetary control

Efficient use of the large expenditure on staffing has become an ever more pressing constraint in the NHS. Many authorities are now operating either locally conceived budgetary control systems or those derived from the Standard Accounting System. An example will illustrate how manpower information can assist both the budget holder and the accountant in controlling manpower expenditure within the limits set by the budget allocation. In the establishment of a budget the staffing requirements must be identified and costed. Classification of staff can be achieved either through the SAS coding which is automatically included on each employee's STAMP record, or through the direct input to STAMP of a local budget code. In this way, all the information held on each individual by STAMP can be produced in a budget classification and, through the use of one of the ad hoc enquiry facilities, can be output regularly in the format required.

The costing of the manpower element to set up a budget can also be facilitated by the use of STAMP data. Instead of simply taking the average of the salary scales involved and adding on a standard cost addition for overtime and other payments made at an enhanced rate, STAMP can provide accurate data on the basic salary (taking into account the different incremental points of employees), and on the amount of overtime, night duty, weekend duty, and other enhanced payments made over the last year to the employees in question. In this way the initial budget allocation is based upon fact rather than upon normative estimates.

Once a budget has been agreed, the budget holder is required to keep within the limits over the financial year. Whilst monthly accounts of expenditure may be provided it is difficult to control it without a detailed knowledge of how the manpower expenses have been incurred. As the STAMP records for each individual hold monthly and cumulative data on all the hours worked and the different payments made for these hours, it is possible for a budget holder to obtain regular monthly reports of this information. Whether ad hoc or standard reports are used the budget holder is able to regulate overtime hours and the number of hours worked at enhanced rates, and can also monitor the validity of the budget originally allocated. High turnover can increase manpower costs because of the need to supervise a high level of inexperienced staff. A factor such as the need to offer day release to junior staff with the subsequent requirement to cover their absence can also inflate expenditure. In addition, a budget holder with only a few staff may find it difficult to cover times of annual leave without the additional expense of employing temporary or agency staff. Such instances can be highlighted through the efficient utilisation of STAMP data.

Another major requirement for managers, and particularly of budget holders, is the need to monitor levels of absence, both planned and unplanned, and to be aware of the implications of absence on manpower expenditure. At the moment STAMP does not have the facility to hold or analyse absence information although this aspect is due to be covered in a future module. (10) Currently, a budget holder must keep manual records of the time lost by the department and has to combine the results of these with the STAMP records to monitor the situation.

Manpower monitoring

There are innumerable ways in which managers in the NHS can improve their understanding of the workforce and begin to actively control the manpower resource. The following examples show some simple ways in which the manpower information available from STAMP could be used to assist in this.

Most authorities, though in varying levels of detail, have drawn up plans for their future requirements for manpower. Whilst it is an easy matter for a local manager to check that appointments have been made as authorised, the further away from the local situation the more difficult it is for authorities to monitor the overall achievement of their manpower plans. Regular monitoring of the changes in staffing levels against the original plans can pinpoint areas where investigation and perhaps even a revision of the plan itself are required. This monitoring can be done in terms of the overall numbers (and wte) of staff employed at regular intervals using whatever classification of staff is required. This is easily derived from STAMP.

In some cases the number of staff in post is not sufficient for monitoring purposes. Often an authority wishes to ensure that the standards of staff cover are adequate and will require regular information on the staff to service ratios. In these cases the STAMP head count data would have to be combined with information from other sources such as the annual bed state return (SH3), or population records, either manually or by the development of a simple programme. This would also provide a useful planning tool if comparisons between different locations were made.

Another simple but illuminating monitoring device is to use the STAMP data to obtain the average costs of different groups of staff and to look at the variations in expenditure across different locations. Often such variation can be explained by such factors as the need to employ more highly graded staff than usual because of the local wage competition with the private sector. In many cases it is less expensive to appoint a new member of staff than to increase overtime of existing employees. The quest for data which will encourage manpower comparisons is similarly illustrated by labour turnover rates. Periodic reports giving comparative turnover and stability indices for similar departments or hospitals in an authority will often enable managers to identify problem areas.

Finally, the calculation of the implications of changes in employment conditions such as pay awards, annual leave entitlements, or reductions in the working week can all be simplified by the use of STAMP. For example, the implications for an authority of an increase in overtime rates or payments for 'unsocial' hours can quickly be generated by examining the number of hours actually worked at the old rates over the past year and uplifting these by the amount awarded.

Training in the use of manpower information

Despite the earlier clamours for more manpower information, as expressed
during the design stage of main STAMP, there is still much uncertainty
about the uses of even the SPS derived information contained in module
one of STAMP. For managers to make full use of manpower information
they must not only be aware of what information is available but also
have some knowledge of manpower planning techniques together with an
understanding of how manpower planning itself contributes to the
planning and management of health services. An essential part of this
process is the ability to extract facts from figures and to know how to
relate manpower information to other available information on service
provision, workload, and expenditure so that managers can ensure the
effective planning and utilisation of their manpower resource.

With the above aims in mind and with the launch of main STAMP planned,
a multidisciplinary group was set up under the direction of the Nuffield
Centre for Health Services Studies, liaising with staff at Wessex, to
produce a training package focusing upon developing and increasing the
awareness of the uses and benefits of manpower information, with STAMP
as one vehicle for obtaining this information. The training package
was in two parts: a general introduction to the STAMP system,
consisting of a guide to its structure, contents, and facilities; and
a set of case studies based on real-life situations concerned with
operational management and planning. The case studies ranged from the
establishment of a budget to the development of manpower guidelines in
the context of a variety of service planning proposals. While the
manpower information in each case study is derived from the STAMP
system, the case studies are self standing. Their general concern is
with developing awareness of manpower information, the use to which it
can be put, and the ability to define the particular information
required in different situations, irrespective of its source. (11)

CONCLUSION

This chapter has attempted to demonstrate how manpower information can
be utilised. Nevertheless, manpower information does not offer the
means for resolving all problems which arise. In practice, even before
STAMP (and its equivalents) became available, there was a considerable
volume of manpower data that attracted little interest or analysis.

The idea of STAMP arose from a more general awareness of the benefits
of better information and of the need to concentrate efforts in its
provision. As technical misgivings were dispelled with the successful
operation of the interim system other arguments were raised so that even
the main system fell far short of users' information requirements. The
initial demands for the development of additional modules to capture and
analyse information such as employee's address, next of kin, hobbies,
qualifications, country of origin, nationality and many others are
lessening as authorities begin to realise the amount of effort that
would be required of themselves and as they begin to question more
deeply how they would use such information.

The increasing demand for training in the field of manpower planning over the last two years has emphasised the fact that few people even know how to make use of the basic payroll information held on STAMP. The recently developed training package has been designed with this in mind. The knowledge of how to use this information is the foundation for successful manpower planning. Without this, the potential of a manpower information system such as STAMP will never be fully exploited. With the introduction of main STAMP, the common remark, even misconception, that manpower planning cannot develop in the NHS because of the lack of an adequate data base can be put to the test.

***** STAFF IN CONFIDENCE *****

STAMP PERSONAL RECORD PRINT AS AT 24/07/80

***** STAFF IN CONFIDENCE *****

SURNAME:- WILSON   FORENAMES:- LINDSAY CHARLOTTE

AUTHORITY:- 99   PAYROLL:- 99   PAYPOINT:- 99   PERSONAL NO:- 99999

ADDRESS:-   9 ELLAND ROAD, FRIMSHAW

DATE OF BIRTH:- 16/01/57   SEX/MARITAL STATUS:- FEMALE/SINGLE

NATIONALITY:- NOT KNOWN   ETHNIC ORIGIN:- NOT KNOWN

STARTING DATES.

IN NHS:-   06/01/80
IN UNIT:-
FOR PAY:-   06/01/80
IN AUTHORITY:-   06/01/81
INCREMENT DUE:-
IN PRESENT GRADE:-

MAIN FINANCIAL CODE:-   00/30/18/24/210131

AREA/DISTRICT:-

PAYSCALE:- N051   POINT ON SCALE:- 00   OCCUPATION CODE:- 130

OCCUPATION DESCRIPTION:-   NURSING ASSTCM ILL)

NATIONAL INSURANCE NO:- YS226616   NAT. INSURANCE LETTER:- D

SUPERANNUATION CODE/CLASS/DIVISION NO:-   011/2/

HOURS/SESSIONS.   * FULL TIME *

CONTRACT:-   40.00   SESSION/HOURLY RATE:-   £1.2040
STANDARD:-   40.00
REPLACEMENT:-   OFFSCALE DIFFERENCE:-

ALLOWANCE AND DEDUCTIONS

CODE	DESCRIPTION	HOURS THIS PERIOD	HOURS TO DATE	VALUE THIS PERIOD	VALUE TO DATE
000	GROSS COST			335.85	335.85
035	PSYCH LEAD			17.62	17.62
922	INCOME TAX			48.45	48.45
924	NAT INSUR			14.62	14.62
A01	BASIC PAY			208.92	208.92
A03	SAT. ENHANCED	22.50	22.50	9.02	9.02
A04	SUN. ENHANCED	29.50	29.50	23.64	23.64
A06	UNSOCIAL HOURS	12.50	12.50	5.01	5.01
A11	WEEKDAY O/T	11.75	11.75	21.49	21.49
B04	SUPERANNUATION			15.77	15.77
B05	EMPLOYER N.I.			30.74	30.74
B06	EMPLOYER SUP.			19.71	19.71

PERSONAL HISTORY RECORDS.   FORMER NAME:-

PAYSCALE:- N051   OCC.CODE:- 130   PT-ON SCALE:- 00
START DATE IN AUTHORITY:- 06/01/80   OLD INCREMENT DATE:- 06/01/81
START DATE IN UNIT:-   PERIOD END DATE:- 30/04/80
START DATE IN GRADE:-
MAIN FINANCIAL CODE:-   02/18/02/50/000000

SURNAME:- WILSON   INITIALS:- LC   PERSONAL NO:- 99999

***** STAFF IN CONFIDENCE *****

SURNAME:- WILSON   INITIALS:- LC   PERSONAL NO:- 99999

***** STAFF IN CONFIDENCE *****

Appendix 1 STAMP Output: Master File Print

EXPERIMENT 6 FOR SALISBURY

ANALYSIS OF STAFF NUMBERS AND TURNOVER BY AGE GROUP

DISTRICT SALISBURY HO   31

HOSPITAL   HOSPITAL UNIT CODE 01   STAFF GROUP QUALIFIED NURSES

AGE OF STAFF
============

TURNOVER OF STAFF
=================

AGE GROUP	PERCENTAGE OF STAFF IN AGE GROUP	% OF ALL	ACT NO.	PERCENTAGE TURNOVER LEVEL	% TRNV	N OF LVRS
<25 YRS	******************	26%	97	<25 *************	28 %	38
25-29	**************	18%	67	25-29 *****************	36 %	38
30-34	*********	10%	38	30-34 ****************	35 %	21
35-39	**********	11%	40	35-39 *******	16 %	8
40-44	*************	15%	55	40-44 ******	15 %	10
45-49	********	09%	33	45-49 *****	10 %	4
50-54	*******	07%	27	50-54 ***	6 %	2
55-59	****	04%	16	55-59 *********	20 %	4
60YRS+	*	01%	3	60YRS+ *********************************	70 %	7

```
    I----I----I----I----I----I----I----I----I
    0   5   10  15  20  25  30  35  40
    PERCENTAGE OF TOTAL STAFF IN POST
```

```
    I----I----I----I----I----I----I----I----I
    0   5   10  15  20  25  30  35  40
    PERCENTAGE OF STAFF LEAVING IN AGE GROUP
```

ANALYSIS OF DATA SHOWN

	< 25	25-29	30-34	35-39	40-44	45-49	50-54	55-59	60+	TOTAL
IN POST	97	67	38	40	55	31	27	16	3	376
LEAVERS	38	38	21	8	10	4	2	4	7	132
TURNOVER %	28 %	36 %	35 %	16 %	15 %	10 %	6 %	20 %	70 %	25 %

TURNOVER IS DEFINED AS THE   NUMBER OF STAFF LEAVING SINCE START OF CURRENT FINANCIAL YEAR   x 100
                             NUMBER OF STAFF AT END OF LAST MONTH + LEAVERS

Appendix 2   STAMP Output: DESIGN-A-FORM

79

NOTES

(1) Data on staff in post at 30 September each year, returned to the DHSS on SBH forms.

(2) North Western Regional Health Authority is the centre of responsibility for SPS.

(3) Cambridge Area Health Authority (Teaching), A Computerised Manpower Information System, King's Fund Project Paper, London 1976.

(4) For a discussion of MAPLIN see, R.Petch, 'The Role of the DHSS', Chapter Six of this volume.

(5) West Midlands Regional Health Authority is the centre of responsibility for SAS.

(6) Possible uses of data such as STAMP produces are outlined in, T.L.Hall and A.Mejia (eds), Health Manpower Planning, World Health Organisation, Geneva 1978, in Table 7, pp.96-98.

(7) MAPLIN Report no.3, 1979, is concerned with the development of a standard categorisation of qualifications.

(8) Full details of Design-A-Form together with instructions for its use are provided in a STAMP User Manual which has been circulated to Regions adopting main STAMP.

(9) For example, there are the MANPLAN packages: see, Civil Service Department, A Management Guide to Manpower Planning Models, HMSO, London 1975; also, the various contributions in Chapter Three of this volume, particularly the one concerned with nursing.

(10) For previous work in this area, see, MAPLIN Report no.2, DHSS, Absence from Work, London 1975, which provides a standard classification scheme.

(11) For a more detailed account of this training package, see, A.F.Long and J.Cree, 'Manpower Information: Case Studies for Training', Health Services Manpower Review, vol.6, no.3, 1980.

5 The Politics of Health Manpower
S. Harrison

'One of the great difficulties . . . is that of reconciling planning and
democracy . . . The freedoms that belong to democracy present themselves
as obstacles to successful planning. The rationality implicit in
planning appears to be an enemy of the sectional pressures unleashed by
democracy.' (1) These words seem to encapsulate the paradox of
manpower planning in an NHS composed of such sectional pressures. The
purposes of this chapter are to show that the NHS has not generally
succeeded in achieving a smooth match of the demand for and supply of
manpower. It illustrates some of the sectional pressures bearing on
this adjustment and the way in which they are presently synthesised,
arguing that in spite of the recent concern for manpower planning in the
Service, they have been insufficiently recognised. The chapter
concludes with a consideration of the possibilities of obtaining a
smoother match from the present arrangements which, it is argued, are
unlikely to undergo substantial change.

In order to state why it is that manpower planning matters anyway it
is necessary to look beyond the simple assertion that labour is one of
the factors of production and needs to be tailored to the intended
product. In fact those who work in the NHS are often able to
determine, in an active sense, the nature of its product. The NHS
constitutes for all practical quantitative purposes the whole of the
UK's health industry, and most of the output of this industry is free
at the point of delivery. The price mechanism is not available to
allocate values and priorities and to adjust demand and supply.
Values have therefore to be allocated politically; planning generally
in the NHS is simply an attempt to do this systematically. Although
national economic performance places ultimate limits on resources
available for health care delivery (since the whole of GNP could not
be allocated in this way) the actual allocation is planned by
governments. And within the global resource figure, distribution is
once again the allocation of values by planning. But planning is not
a technical process, rather a highly subjective one, a point concealed
by the quotation which opens this chapter. In spite of their
technical complexity, the RAWP and analogous formulae for Scotland and
Wales are themselves 'partly a matter of subjective judgement and
political decision.' (2) Where the market is not available for
allocation, planning is a political process.

The first reason for the importance of planning manpower is simply that manpower represents a very large proportion of the resources of the Service; three-quarters of the expenditure of the NHS goes on salaries and wages. A second reason however is that it is difficult to think of an organisation whose staff have a greater role in the design of the 'product' than occurs in the NHS. Indeed, in the absence of more than generalised definitions of 'health', health workers virtually define the product and the need at which it is aimed. This is of course particularly, though not exclusively, true of doctors as 'leaders of the health care team and the primary decision makers in the health care industry. Their decisions to treat patients commit resources such as nurses, technicians, equipment and materials.' (3) Thus the mix and varieties of workers employed in the NHS are prime determinants of the nature of the health service delivered.

It is almost a commonplace that the NHS has failed successfully to match demand for and supply of manpower. The first dimension of this failure is the geographical distribution of trained NHS workers, the inequity of which is illustrated by data presented in the Report of the Royal Commission on the NHS. (4) The second dimension relates to the numbers in which health workers exist, and is best illustrated by examples of controversy and precipitate change in the supply of three particular professions.

The first of these, doctors, may fairly be described as a long-running epic since it dates back over 20 years. In 1957 the Willink Committee (5) recommended, on the basis of the then age structure of the profession and other factors, a cut of 10 per cent in the intake of medical students. However, by 1961 the Platt Report (6) was recommending an increase in numbers of consultants and hence of doctors in training; the then Minister of Health, Mr. Enoch Powell, agreed for an increase of 10 per cent. It was pointed out in 1974 that 'every group that has studied hospital medical staffing in the last 20 years (has) recommended further expansion of the Consultant grade.' (7) More recently 'in one of those sudden mass conversions usually associated with religious revivalism, it has become accepted almost overnight that Britain faces an impending surplus of doctors.' (8) However the Merrison Report concludes 'that the planned output of medical graduates is about right.' (9)

In contrast to doctors, conventional wisdom concerning the supply of nurses remained unchanged from 1945 (10) for 30 years: there was a shortage. In 1976, however, there arose 'widespread fears of a glut of nurses. In reaction, trainee numbers were cut back, those qualifying were warned that they could not be guaranteed employment, and older nurses were prepared for early retirement.' (11) A further change of opinion followed swiftly so that by 1977 health authorities were reporting difficulties in nurse recruitment. Authorities were subsequently encouraged by DHSS to reconsider their reduced intakes of trainees.

The third example of precipitate reaction concerns radiographers whose numbers, along with many other professional and technical groups, grew consistently from 1948 onwards, accelerating more recently. In 1975 the Halsbury Committee (12) identified a 25 per cent shortage but by early 1977 there were reports that some newly qualifying students would be unable to be found posts in the hospitals or localities in which they had undergone training.   In response, the intake of students for October 1977 was reduced to two-thirds of the former permitted level. In spite of a decision that the restriction will remain for the time being, there are reports (13) that the new level will quickly result in shortages.   In any event given that diagnostic tests rather than the number of patients treated have typified the recent past use by the NHS of increased resources, it seems unlikely that there is any probability of radiographer unemployment.

The three examples chosen - doctors, nurses and radiographers - are only the more extreme examples of a manpower system which has been characterised by an inability to achieve a long term coincidence of demand and supply.   In contrast to what has been described above it might be expected, *a priori*, that the NHS would find it easier to plan manpower successfully than any other organisation of comparable size. The reasoning underlying this is that the state has established a virtual monopoly as employer of medical and related skills, and is therefore relatively immune from the operations of labour markets.   In other words, given a knowledge of future service developments and a reasonable forecast of labour turnover, 'the NHS has . . . an opportunity of securing a match in supply and demand which is rare in the UK manpower economy.' (14)   What then are the reasons underlying the lack of success which has been demonstrated?   One reason is that the management arrangements for the NHS are not, unlike the Civil Service, monolithic;   each health authority is a legal employer in its own right, reaching many of its own planning decisions and determining many of its own employment policies.   Hence, central decisions do not entirely determine manpower need nor, as is discussed below, supply.

A more far reaching reason for the difficulty of successful manpower planning is that this fragmentation of decision making extends beyond health authorities to other groups and to individuals.   People, in spite of the application to them of the objectified term 'manpower', are not a passive resource but have interests of their own which conflict with those of the planners.   These interests may relate to individuals, who might object to physical transfer, changes in working times or duties, or to groups, whether defined by profession, status, place in the organisation structure, or other characteristic.   It is for instance almost part of the definition of a craft or profession that it seeks so far as possible to be self governing and to prevent in particular dilution or over supply of practitioners.   In the words of recent analysts of the medical profession 'occupational strategies are generated in the attempt to reduce uncertainty and obtain a high degree of control over market forces.' (15)   This may not coincide with the planner's view of what is rational, but is certainly rational from the point of view of the professional.   The conflict of interest over numbers of professionals is frankly expressed by Klein who points out that 'a surplus of doctors will bring down the relative level of medical salaries and thus make it possible to employ more doctors;   an outcome which, though clearly repugnant to existing members of the profession, will benefit the public as a whole.' (16)   There may also be individual differences;   for instance many doctors would prefer to see expansion occur in the more prestigious specialties, which equate roughly with those where there is no shortage.   This conflicts with such current planning priorities as the long stay services. (17)   There may also be conflict within a profession, for instance, as to whether the ratio of consultant to junior hospital posts should be increased.

It is clear that similar conflict can exist over geography. A planner may consider it desirable that acute services be centralised in a new district general hospital or may wish to encourage the movement of dietitians away from teaching hospitals. Such plans are not likely to coincide with the travel preferences of the individuals involved. Thus, although the NHS may apparently tend towards monopoly, it is widely dispersed, and in the absence of the direction of labour the employment of the desired number of particular staff will not guarantee their being in the required location. (18)

Contrary to what might have been expected manpower planning for the NHS is not especially straightforward. In addition, the attitude of planners in the Service is not fully attuned to the centrality of human resources as service constraints; there are still capital developments in progress which will prove difficult to staff as a result of labour market forces rather than financial ones. (19) The historical tendency to think of planning in terms of buildings, services and equipment in that order and only fourthly of staff will not disappear quickly, in spite of the sharp reduction of capital as a proportion of health authority expenditure which has occurred since 1974. This reduction seems likely to continue in view of Britain's economic prospects and government commitment to reduce public expenditure. The extent to which the NHS can continue to develop without reallocating resources seems limited, and health authorities who wish to do other than allow their services to stagnate will be forced increasingly to consider reallocation of resources; planning is likely to become an even more difficult process when it seeks to make inroads into the status quo. This is not to say that no progress in NHS manpower planning has been made. Other chapters in this book analyse some of the current initiatives. It is notable that much of this progress has been centred on the gathering of information and related activities. Whilst such collection is logically prior it is hoped that it will not become a proxy for genuine attempts to match demand and supply. The next section of this chapter is concerned to analyse the way in which demand for NHS labour is generated by attempting to list and briefly discuss the demand factors, commencing with staffing norms.

There are in operation in the Service a very large number of norms and guides to manning levels in particular circumstances. These vary very greatly in sophistication from data based upon work study or patient dependency, through guidance issued by professional organisations and official minimum standards, to simple indices and rules of thumb at the opposite extreme. (20) The one feature which these share is the appearance of objectivity built, often very carefully, upon a subjective basis. (21) These norms therefore actually constitute value judgements about how resources ought to be allocated. The fact of the co-existence of a range of differing norms (perhaps local, regional and national) for the same set of circumstances stands in testimony of this since a 'truly objective' norm, if there could be such a thing, could not be contradicted. These can be used to provide an 'illusion of neutrality . . . thereby avoiding confrontation with the true political nature of . . . decisions (to rationalise services).' (22) They have no sanctity and will tend to be mobilised in arguments in support of an

objective already identified, rather than as a means of determining
objectives.   This process can occur in, though is by no means confined
to, discussions between health authorities where, say, a Regional Health
Authority has the right to grant or withhold the establishment of
particular new posts.   This may be referred to as 'hierarchical
discretion'.

The activities of interest groups within the NHS are major
determinants of manpower demand.   The term can equally be understood to
refer to groups within or outside a health authority; such groups may
be different management or professional groups, or management and staff
groups.   This might be characterised as 'local bargaining', something
which has occurred for many years between management and professional
groups but which is now beginning to include trade unions, reflecting
the growth of union membership and local industrial relations activity
over the last 10 years.   Other relevant factors are the requirements of
the DHSS planning system that plans be the subject of consultation with
staff interests, the obligation that staff be consulted on proposed
hospital closures, and the enactment of provisions for the disclosure to
trade unions of information for collective bargaining purposes. (23)
All these, as well as health and safety legislation, can be expected to
increase the extent to which manning levels, for both existing and
developing on projected services, are outside the area of unilateral
management decision making.

Another determinant of demand is national collective bargaining.
Whilst this may not in itself exert a major influence on the numbers of
staff sought for NHS employment, from time to time issues such as a
reduction in the standard weekly hours of work certainly do. (24)
Probably of more significance however is the fact that role definitions
for NHS occupations are often contained in Whitley agreements.   It is
obvious that the question of role is inseparable from the issue of the
number and description of staff required for the delivery of a specific
health care service.   As will be seen in a later section of this
chapter, Whitley Councils are not the only bodies involved in role
definition.   Such definition is itself an important component of supply
in that it determines the nature of some of the manpower which is
supplied.   As has been observed already, knowledge of what will be
supplied can modify what is demanded.

Pressure groups representing health service consumers, or sections of
them, have become increasingly prominent in recent years and 'have
achieved some successes' (25) in influencing the provision of services,
and therefore on health authority staffing requirements.   These groups
include Community Health Councils (CHCs), some of which have adopted a
proactive role in pressing for service provisions and which in any event
have the right to be consulted on plans and proposed closures.   There
are also other groups such as MIND, Age Concern, the National
Association for the Welfare of Children in Hospital, and the Patients'
Association.   It seems doubtful if the effects procured by these
groups, or CHCs, approach the results of action by NHS producer groups.

A further determinant of demand is the precise nature of the local
interface between health and social service provision.   It is clear
that the nature and extent of local social service provision for, say,
the elderly bear heavily upon the need for geriatric beds and

appropriate hospital staff. The nature of this interface will normally be stable but could on occasions change radically; for instance, following cutbacks in social service provision consequent on the present government policies for reductions in local authority spending.

Related to the above issue of substitutability of services as between authorities is that of staff substitution, either the establishment of new grades of worker or the transfer of work between existing grades. (26) These are only partly resolved by Whitley Council requirements. Extra-Whitley national industrial relations factors, as well as local bargaining, may be the prime determinants. An example of such a resolution is the continued opposition by the medical profession (except for the brief period in which medical assistant posts were created) to the creation of a sub-consultant grade recommended by the Guillebaud Committee in 1956, the Platt Working Party in 1961 and the Todd Commission in 1968. (27)

Another form of possible substitution is that of capital equipment for labour. Because health care services are personal services it is virtually impossible to reduce labour intensity at the point of health care delivery. Indeed the history of technology in the NHS is such that labour intensity has probably increased with some developments. The opportunity exists to substitute capital for labour in support services activities; laundries, pathology laboratories and central sterile supplies departments can be automated and new hospital designs may require lower manning levels than do older buildings. However, as Engleman has pointed out, 'new hospitals do not simply replicate the services of old ones, but tend to expand and improve them. Consequently, while they may be more efficient, the cost of the new mix of services will tend to outweigh the cost savings arising out of the replacement of an inefficient capital stock.' (28) This is equally true of laundry or laboratory automation. Technology also affects the division of NHS labour and has probably contributed to the proliferation of grades of health worker since the NHS's inception.

Finance as a determinant of (or perhaps more accurately as a constraint upon) demand has been left until last since it is, in total at least, all pervasive with regard to the other determinants. There is a clear and only marginally negotiable limit to the financial resources allocated by one level in the management hierarchy to the next lower level. Within this parameter and assuming that funds are not 'earmarked', the other determinants of demand can operate freely and in relation to whatever determinants of demand exist for resources other than labour. The exception is where some specific negative external control, such as the recent 'standstill' on management and administrative posts, exists. Thus budgetary considerations do not of themselves determine the demand for any particular group of staff.

It may be objected that items such as population, health care 'need', morbidity, and mortality have not been included here as determinants of health manpower demand. Such objections may be answered in two ways. Firstly, such factors are often contained in the determinants which have been discussed. Hence population is often a component of staffing norms, and measures of ill health might be taken into account in the formulation of health authorities' plans. Secondly, there is no evidence that health authorities situated in areas of low morbidity make more modest manpower demands than those where the need is apparently greater. (29)

An attempt has been made in Figure 5.1 to summarise the foregoing analysis of demand and to relate it to supply. The scheme is generalised and can be applied at any level of the NHS, particularly the operational planning level. It applies equally to particular staff groups or to the workforce as a whole. The horizontal axis emphasises what, for an employing authority, is the centrality of its existing workforce and any changes, either reductions or increases, which it intends to make. The shift from the status quo is made, at least theoretically, via plans (Arrow A). However, recognition that in practice many service changes are not formally planned, or are even unplanned, is found in the alternative direct connection (Arrow B). (30) Demand for and supply of labour, at the top and bottom respectively of the figure, affect the maintenance of the existing workforce (Arrows C and D); in the case of changes the effect may be allowed for in plans (Arrows E and F) or may lead directly to the changes (Arrows G and H). Finally, knowledge of the supply situation may help to determine demand (Arrow I), and vice versa.

This section turns to the question of supply. Whilst the general relationship of supply to other factors is indicated in Figure 5.1, no attempt was made to analyse its determinants, which may be roughly divided into external and internal factors. External factors relate primarily to labour markets and are dealt with here rather briefly on the grounds that whilst they may be predicted by planners, most cannot be modified to any significant extent. One, often unnoticed, of these is demography. It has been shown that over the next 10 years the future 'supply of nurses will be under pressure from the likely problems in recruitment and retention', (31) due to the twin factors that by 1988 the number of persons in the population aged 18 - the typical age for entry to nurse training - will have declined by 12 per cent, and that 41 per cent of present nurses are in the prime reproductive ages and therefore relatively highly likely to leave nursing for family responsibilities.

More easily visible are the current level of unemployment in areas where recruitment is sought and the level of female activity rates: indeed, health services in Europe 'depend on three women for every man.' (32) Not all groups of health workers can be regarded as part of the same market, since markets may be subdivided along lines of both skill and geography; thus professionals are unlikely to seek work elsewhere than in their profession whilst manual or clerical groups may well seek work with a variety of types of employer. So far as geography is concerned, it is clear that the latter groups will tend to change employment within a limited local area (probably daily travelling distance. On the other hand doctors, senior administrators and senior managers in other disciplines will often be prepared to seek employment and promotion over much of Great Britain. No doubt there could also be said to exist between these extremes what might be termed a regional labour market, but it is less clear what staff groups might be involved. Other supply factors related to geography include the rural or urban nature of the workplace location and traditional habits of mobility and travel to work patterns, often as reinforced by the local provision of

Fig 5.1 *A model of Labour demand and supply.*

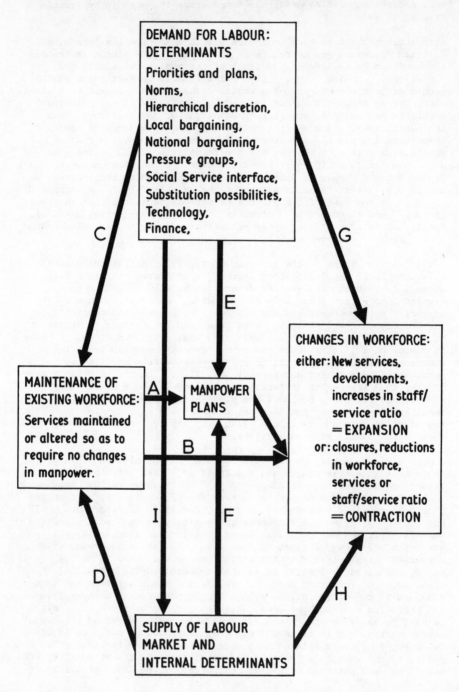

DEMAND FOR LABOUR:
DETERMINANTS
Priorities and plans,
Norms,
Hierarchical discretion,
Local bargaining,
National bargaining,
Pressure groups,
Social Service interface,
Substitution possibilities,
Technology,
Finance,

C

G

E

MAINTENANCE OF
EXISTING WORKFORCE:
Services maintained
or altered so as to
require no changes
in manpower.

A

MANPOWER
PLANS

B

CHANGES IN WORKFORCE:
either: New services,
developments,
increases in staff/
service ratio
= EXPANSION
or: closures, reductions
in workforce,
services or
staff/service ratio
= CONTRACTION

I

F

D

H

SUPPLY OF LABOUR
MARKET AND
INTERNAL DETERMINANTS

public transport.   Also relevant can be the social class structure of
the area surrounding a workplace;   there are examples of hospitals
situated in commuter areas which have found it impossible to recruit
domestic staff.

Immigration and emigration have a part to play, especially in the case
of health professionals.   It is widely recognised, for instance, that
'the dependence of the NHS on the inflow of doctors from overseas has
been considerable', (33) and this is not only true for doctors.   The
question of emigration has been and still is contentious, though the
numbers by no means approach the numbers of immigrants.   Both
emigration and immigration will have to be considered by planners in the
light of British membership of the European Economic Community and the
free movement of labour which it allows.   Labour supply is also
affected by the ordinary course of turnover due to such factors as
retirement, pregnancy, job changes and dismissals.

Relative levels of pay are often argued to be of prime importance so
far as the supply of labour is concerned.   It is beyond doubt that low
relative pay has in the past been associated with difficulties in
recruitment of ancillary staff and perhaps also of nurses.   However, in
the case of the NHS professions, status and the vocational feelings of
entrants to them are important.   It has further been pointed out that
although those negotiating medical salaries have tended to argue that
increases in these are necessary to attract suitable recruits into the
profession, 'in fact . . . well qualified young people apply in large
numbers for admission to medical schools and are also rejected in large
numbers.   In recent years medicine has been the most popular subject to
study at university if the ratio of applicants to places is taken into
the appropriate measure.' (34)   It is also doubtful whether those
considering entry to NHS professions have very much knowledge about
their eventual earnings.   It is, for instance, difficult to believe
that someone applying for nurse training has any accurate information
about the earnings likely to accrue after qualification.   This casts
doubt, so far as such professions are concerned, on the directness of
the relationship between pay and recruitment.

It also seems likely that the levels of pay of NHS workers, like many
other workers, are determined to a large extent by convention.
Evidence of this may be found in the importance attached by Whitley
Councils to the 'complex system of linkages between the rates
negotiated on behalf of groups of NHS staff and rates negotiated for
other groups elsewhere' and the 'system of internal linkage between
groups of staff within the NHS.' (35)   In addition, ad hoc pay
enquiries feature frequently: the Clegg Commission reports on
ancillary, ambulance and nursing staffs.   All this points to little
attempt on the part of those responsible for NHS manpower policies to
attempt to counter shortages by making employment more financially
attractive.   It is worth noting that where substantial pay awards have
been made as a result of ad hoc enquiries, they have been constituted in
response to major political or industrial relations issues.   'The
ability and willingness of the NHS to respond to labour market
pressures . . . is clearly constrained.' (36)

It follows from much of the above discussion that the number of
places available for persons to train for work in the NHS is a crucial

determinant of supply. This factor is clearly not one which can be
considered external or relating to labour markets but forms the
substance of what are termed internal supply determinants. One
preliminary point which needs to be made is that the number entering
training is neither the same as the number who qualify nor the number
who eventually practise: there is a 'drop-out' or failure rate which
intervenes. (37) The short term importance of the availability of
training places is further moderated by the length of the training
itself, a lag which, incidentally, weakens the connection between levels
of remuneration of trained staff and the number of persons applying for
training.

Nevertheless the number of training places available for each NHS
occupational group remains a major determinant of the level of supply of
that group. An attempt to identify the variables which in turn
determine the number of training places is made in Figure 5.2. In
order to allow depiction of the extremes, the concept of training places
has been extended to include non professional occupations for whom the
number of training places is in practice simply identical to the number
of vacancies for the basic grade of the occupation. The essence of
Figure 5.2 is that it represents a conceptual continuum indicating the
number of institutions involved in the determination of the number of
training places available for broad groups of NHS occupations. The
stress on institutions springs from the impracticability of generalising
about intra-institutional factors; thus an NHS employing authority is
considered for this purpose as one factor in spite of the probability
that it will contain within itself several different shades of opinion
and a number of interest subgroupings. The continuum therefore
illustrates at its left hand extreme the situation where the number of
training places is determined by one organisation only, the employing
authority itself. The groups of staff to which this situation applies
are those whose training is 'on the job', that is the majority of
ancillary and clerical staff. It may be objected that some members of
these groups, especially administrative and secretarial staff, do
receive education and/or training off the job. The point is however
that such training is not a prerequisite of entry to a practising post
in that occupation. For this reason, national staff committees do not
appear in Figure 5.2. Movement towards the right hand end of the
continuum indicates an increase in the number of institutions involved.
Broad staff groups have been located on the continuum and it is possible
in principle to locate any specific staff group in the same way.
Beneath each broad group an attempt has been made to list the
institutions (in each case in addition to the employing authority)
significantly involved in supply determination. It will be noted that
some of those listed are more concerned with defining the role and
training requirements of staff groups than the numbers, but, as has
already been argued, it is unrealistic to separate the two issues. It
will also be evident that the direction of influence on labour supply by
many of the institutions is towards its restriction.

Figure 5.2 may be further explained by reference to three specific
occupations, those used earlier in this paper as examples of contention
over manpower requirements; nurses, radiographers and doctors. The
case of nursing is quite straightforward since not only are schools of
nursing located in Districts or Areas but are directed by employees of
the health authority, which also employs the students and pupils, who

Fig 5.2 *A Model of Training Places* (a)

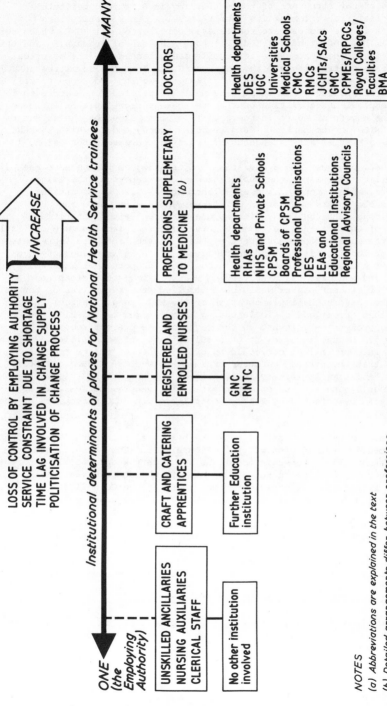

LOSS OF CONTROL BY EMPLOYING AUTHORITY
SERVICE CONSTRAINT DUE TO SHORTAGE
TIME LAG INVOLVED IN CHANGE SUPPLY
POLITICISATION OF CHANGE PROCESS

INCREASE

MANY

DOCTORS

Health departments
DES
UGC
Universities
Medical Schools
CMC
RMCs
JCHTs/SACs
GMC
CPMEs/RPGCs
Royal Colleges/
Faculties
BMA
DDRB

PROFESSIONS SUPPLEMETARY
TO MEDICINE *(b)*

Health departments
RHAs
NHS and Private Schools
CPSM
Boards of CPSM
Professional Organisations
DES
LEAs and
Educational Institutions
Regional Advisory Councils

REGISTERED AND
ENROLLED NURSES

GNC
RNTC

CRAFT AND CATERING
APPRENTICES

Further Education
institution

UNSKILLED ANCILLARIES
NURSING AUXILIARIES
CLERICAL STAFF

No other institution
involved

Institutional determinants of places for National Health Service trainees

ONE
(the
Employing
Authority)

NOTES
(a) Abbreviations are explained in the text
(b) Detailed arrangements differ between professions,
    the figure is intended to give a broad indication.

91

because of the structure of nurse training in Britain constitute a substantial proportion of its labour force. Other institutions involved in the process are the General Nursing Council (GNC) which sets the syllabus and standards and 'licenses' the school of nursing and the hospitals to which students and pupils are attached for the practical components of training and the Regional Nurse Training Committee (RNTC) which funds to authorities the salaries of teaching and support staff in schools of nursing. It might reasonably be concluded therefore that while employing authorities exert a reasonably high level of influence over the number of nurse learners this is constrained by the extent to which RNTCs are prepared to fund teaching posts, and to which the GNC remains satisfied with standards of training and ward supervision.

However, changes in the education and training of nurses have been a probability ever since the publication of the report of the Briggs Committee which proposed the establishment of colleges of nursing responsible to Area Education Committees whose writ would run coterminous with the boundaries of one or more health authorities. The effect of this may not be to make nurse manpower planning more difficult since the same report lays great emphasis on the 'adequate represent-ation of local attitudes and sufficiently intimate knowledge of local problems and opportunities' and on the need for personnel management and integrated manpower planning. (38) However, it is not clear how the number of student places would be controlled (the report was of course completed before the implementation of the NHS Reorganisation) and it seems that the effect of implementing Briggs might be to shift the nursing profession somewhat to the right of its present location on Figure 5.2 by the involvement of a multiplicity of authorities. In the longer run, any ill effect could be offset by other Briggs recommend-ations that the pattern of nurse training be centred around one basic course, and the flexibility in the use of manpower which this should encourage. The future form of training for general nurses will no doubt also be affected by British compliance with EEC Directives on the subject.

The second example, that of radiographers, falls into the Professions Supplementary to Medicine group in Figure 5.2. They are trained in schools normally located in hospitals and undertake practical experience in working radiology departments whilst receiving DHSS funded bursaries. The Radiographers Board of the Council for Professions Supplementary to Medicine (CPSM), recognises only one qualification for state registration, the Diploma of the College of Radiographers, and has the statutory authority to recognise training institutions and courses of training leading to the diploma. The College and Society of Radiographers are the product of a formal split between the educational and collective bargaining roles respectively of the former Society which occurred in 1978. The two bodies continue to share the same premises and it is not possible to be in membership of one without the other, a joint fee being payable.

The College of Radiographers specifies guidelines in terms of staff, facilities and maximum permitted student intakes to schools of radiography and it was by revision of these that the 1977 reduction in the number of radiography students was achieved. Hence the College/ Society has effective unilateral control over the maximum number of students trained each year. Although in theory the Council and Board

could recognise other qualifying bodies, the composition of the Board -
a majority of radiographers are in practice College members - makes this
unlikely.   In addition, the highly technological requirements of
radiographer training make a change to other institutions impractical.

It should be recognised however that except for the example given in
the preceding paragraph the professions have not generally exploited the
potential power which the training and registration arrangements seem to
offer.   Indeed, it is known that the CPSM is concerned with service
needs and that localised arrangements exist for schools of radiography
and other professions to be to some extent responsive to the needs of
employing authorities who provide practical attachments.

The institutions listed in the relevant section of Figure 5.2 are
intended to give a general indication in respect of all the professions
supplementary to medicine.   Hence Local Education Authorities (LEAs)
are involved in providing student grants in cases where schools are not
located in hospitals. (39)   In considering the role of the CPSM the
historical influence of the medical profession in setting parameters for
practice of the supplementary professions, and the extent of its
representation on the CPSM and its Board should not be forgotten.

The final example, doctors, illustrates well how governments in
practice delegate decision making to, or share it with, other
interested groups.   In theory 'the Government controls the number of
medical school places in Universities' (40) whereas a recent book
concludes that in practice 'medical manpower has remained very much in
control of the medical profession.' (41)   The number of medical under-
graduates is controlled rather indirectly through the Department of
Education of Science (DES) and University Grants Committee (UGC), the
latter allocating resources between the various universities;   although
each university is nominally free to allocate resources between
different academic areas as it sees fit, in practice UGC strategies are
adhered to.   In the case of medicine the relevant strategy emanates
from the DHSS, having originated with the Todd Commission.   Basic
standards for medical practice are determined by the General Medical
Council (GMC).

However, it is insufficient merely to consider the number of medical
students since the number and roles of doctors in the career grades are
also partly determined by the requirements of postgraduate medical
education and the pattern of both training and career posts available.
The Central and Regional Manpower Committees (CMC, RMCs) and RHAs are
involved in the allocation of posts to particular specialities and to
particular regions and areas, whereas the Royal Colleges and Faculties
are able to accredit posts as adequate for training for the appropriate
speciality.   The CMC is thus concerned with the crucial issues of the
distribution of doctors as between career and junior posts as well as
geographically and between specialities.   Accreditation of Senior
Registrar posts and occupants is now largely undertaken by Joint
Committees on Higher Training (JCHTs) and their specialist Advisory
Committees (SACs).   Co-ordination of postgraduate medical education is
the responsibility of the Councils for Postgraduate Medical Education
and Regional Postgraduate Committees (RPGCs).

Finally, the activities of those institutions involved in formal

collective bargaining on behalf of doctors - the BMA and the Doctors'
and Dentists' Review Body (DDRB) - need to be included since the
distribution of medical earnings and the format of doctors' contracts
can affect the shape of the profession especially as between general and
hospital practice.   The BMA also has representation in a number of the
institutions described in the preceding paragraph.   In fact the whole
mechanism is not nearly as pluralistic as the mere listing of the bodies
involved may convey;   not only is the medical profession dominant within
most of them but the same sections of the profession (notably the
Colleges and Faculties) are represented within many.   Nevertheless, the
plurality of institutions does seem to be a barrier to anyone wishing to
plan change.   A senior medical officer from DHSS has pointed out that
'nine out of every ten doctors in active practice work for the National
Health Service and in a sense the Department of Health is their
corporate employer;   yet the Department has no say in the selection of
medical students or the content of medical education.' (42)   It is not
surprising that a recent official publication on medical manpower is
entirely based on the assumption that the nature of the doctor's role
will remain unchanged. (43)

The continuum in Figure 5.2 illustrates the growth in the number of
institutions involved in determining the number of training places for
NHS workers, as one moves from those occupations on the left of the
figure towards the right.   This continuum, however, also represents
variables other than the number of institutions involved.   From the
point of view of the employing authority (and its planners) movement
towards the right of the figure represents an increasing loss of control
over the supply of its labour, and therefore a potentially increasing
constraint on the implementation of its service plans.   Secondly, and
related to this, is the increasing extent to which (moving still from
left to right) individual members of the particular staff groups are
likely to be key figures.   This is not intended to be an argument that
doctors are more important than nurses, or any similar comparison, but
merely that the constraints placed upon health care delivery by a
shortage of a single member of a staff group located to the right of the
continuum are likely to be greater than those caused by a shortage of
someone from the groups located to the left. (44)   A third variable
which approximates to the continuum is length of training for staff
groups.   In conjunction with the number of institutions involved in
each case, this becomes a reasonably accurate indicator of the time lag
involved in changing the number of available training places.

Finally, the continuum might also be held to measure the extent to
which changing the supply of a group of staff is a political process;
the relative importance of market factors decreases with movement
towards the right.   The term political can be understood as relating to
'the activity by which differing interests within a given unit of rule
are conciliated by giving them a share in power.' (45)   So the process
of changing the supply of NHS workers may be a more, or less, political
one.   However, when one turns back to the determinants of demand for
NHS labour analysed earlier in this chapter it is evident that they are
without exception political in nature.   This includes an express view
of financial factors as political rather than economic or technical on
the dual grounds that they are only a constraint at an aggregate level
and that formulae for resource allocation themselves constitute
political statements.   It is clearly not appropriate in a generalised

94

analysis of this kind to place relative weights on the factors
identified as relevant to the determination of manpower levels.
However, if all the demand determinants and a variable but substantial
proportion of the supply determinants are political in nature, it seems
reasonable to characterise the labour supply process as political.
Recognition of this is of particular importance to planners in the NHS
since, it will be recalled, the bulk of labour market or external
determinants of supply are only barely susceptible to planners'
influence.

It is one of the arguments of this chapter that the political nature
of manpower determination in the NHS has received insufficient
recognition.   In practice much of the recent work on the subject has
been heavily biased towards the technical and quantitative.   If the
nature of the process has gone largely unrecognised (though more likely
simply unarticulated) what is the value of quantitative methods into
which so much effort has recently been placed?   Such methods are
important and it is not the purpose of this chapter to suggest that any
of the present developments are not to be welcomed.   The value of
quantitative methods including work study and related techniques lies in
assisting the parties involved in the process of determining manpower
demand and supply to set their own objectives, to assemble arguments
which point to those objectives and to predict the outcome of particular
strategies.   Thus there are pressing needs for data about existing
manpower stock so that there is at least some common ground from which
argument can commence.   Such information can also be used to predict
demand arising from labour turnover.   Knowledge of the cost of
particular strategies allows, in theory at least, calculation of 'the
price of any social demand in terms of relinquished alternatives.' (46)
The importance of such information and the methods for handling it are
great, so long as their use is accompanied by a recognition that they
cannot themselves provide a 'right' answer to the question of which and
how many staff are required for a particular purpose.   It will be
readily seen that the same conclusions apply to other kinds of data and
their use in the broader context of planning.   It follows from what has
been said that the mere production and presentation of data will achieve
nothing;   the conclusion that 'manpower planning is fundamentally a
quantitative process' (47) is unwarranted.   In practice, data is used
selectively to lend support to particular stances.   Unfortunately, the
tendency to assume a single rationality and to treat data as neutral
remains, and can be seen in statements such as 'available criteria and
data are not sufficiently valid and complete to ensure that questions of
occupational structure and work allocation are approached with
sufficient objectivity.' (48)   In practice 'techniques are weak where
opinion, consent, (and) motivation . . . are involved.' (49)

The issue which remains is how manpower planning can become more
effective, and much of the discussion which follows could be applied to
NHS planning in general.   However, since planners and producers may
have very different rationalities, contrasting interpretations of what
is 'effective' arise.   This is not to deny that there are some issues,
for example unemployment among health professionals, which might be
perceived as a common problem.   If it were assumed that health
authorities, and planners on their behalf, ought to determine plans and
implement them, the answer would be that planning would be more
effective if such authorities were more powerful.   In manpower planning

terms this would mean that they would have greater freedom to determine the manpower consequences of their plans and greater control (other than market factors) over the labour supply. However, there is no particular reason to make the initial assumption. Reference is frequently made to the indeterminacy of health care outcomes; neither is there any firm evidence of a consensus as to what is understood by health nor that health authorities are especially in touch with the opinions of their population. Even were the assumption to be granted, it is difficult to see how more power could in practice be exercised. Formal relationships could of course be changed but this may not necessarily make significant changes in the balance of power. Quite apart from the difficulties in devolving to the local level responsibility for professions numbering in total only a few thousand or less, there is no observable trend to indicate other than that professionalism and the present sophisticated division of labour in the NHS will remain. This in itself may ensure that producer groups will continue to figure largely in the process of demand and, especially, supply determination.

It might be asked at this point whether there is a role for planning at all, and whether the political process should simply be allowed to take its course. Such a view seems unwarranted since there are a number of ways in which planning can perform valuable functions. It encourages longer term thinking; it indicates inter-relationships between issues and improves co-ordination; and it helps to identify options for objectives. It serves also as a standard against which the achievement of objectives can be assessed. Although 'planning without political support is no more than an academic exercise . . . politics without planning is usually irrelevant to the needs and aspirations of society.' (50)

If planning of manpower is to continue, how can it be more effective in smoothing out the process of matching supply and demand? It is clear that it will have to become consciously a part of the political system if plans are to have any effect upon events. This points to a negotiating or bargaining role for planners, involving them in the acquisition of the relevant skills. Such skills include analytical and predictive ability along with appropriate contextual knowledge. The role would involve 'identifying the individuals or groups actually or potentially concerned with the problem, the likely reasons for their concern and the solutions they propose, the strength they can mobilise to further their views and the possible points of compromise.' (51) It may be that planners or managers would see the appellations 'political' or 'bargaining' as pejorative, or that they would consider themselves insufficiently powerful for such a role. It might be more appropriate to speak of a 'diplomatic' role. Keeling's concept of the diplomatic system is relevant since it tells much about the attributes likely to be of value to a manpower planner working in such a context. These include knowledge of quantitative methods and the ability to use them in argument, negotiating skills, flexibility and 'the ability to keep a variety of middle-term strategies in a meaningful relationship to long-term objectives while continuing to be concerned in detail with the immediate interface between these strategies and (those affected by them).' (52)

The question arises of who is best placed to carry out such manpower planning. The two aspects of this question are the interests and disciplines which should be involved, and the hierarchical level at which it should be effected.   So far as the first aspect is concerned it seems clear that all whose interests are at stake and all from whom commitment to the eventual outcome is sought should be involved in the process.   In practice, it should not be separated from service planning, requires a multidisciplinary management approach, and should include representatives able so far as possible to commit themselves on behalf of the interest groups (primarily staff) involved.   The second aspect, that of hierarchical level, is less straightforward since it is clear from Figure 5.2 that power is exerted at different levels in respect of different staff groups.   From the point of view of the employing authority there is a shift from bargaining inside the authority to bargaining outside it, with movement towards the right hand end of the continuum.   At present, health authorities have to accept, in respect of some groups of professional staff, the results of bargaining among other institutions.

It is partly a combination of this observation and the independent status of health authorities which has led to various suggestions for the establishment of some kind of centralised NHS manpower commission, (53) though its advocates have not always been clear about its projected role, and there would seem a danger of merely adding a further institution to an already complex process.   The Royal Commission did not accept the suggestion and at the time of writing there is no sign of government support for it.   Whatever the outcome, however, it is not likely that such a commission could serve as anything other than an information centre (a function already partly performed by DHSS), and, if suitably composed, a forum for bargaining to take place.   The latter could help the process to occur more smoothly, but 'the hope that (manpower planning) will replace bargaining is an idle dream.' (54)

To summarise, this chapter has attempted to show that the NHS is a pluralistic and political environment where manpower planning, if it is to influence events, must adopt appropriate political methods.   The chapter has not sought to be prescriptive, but rather analytical;   its conclusions are not radical but consist of ways in which the process as it stands can be influenced.   The status quo is assessed as a powerful force and probable changes to the process as no more than marginal. More radical changes are desirable, but seem unlikely to occur.

The NHS is pluralistic only in the sense that a number of groups and interests are powerful enough to require conciliation.   It is emphatically not pluralistic in a more precise sense of power being non-cumulatively distributed across all groups concerned with the Service.   Indeed, many of the institutions involved in the determin-ation of labour supply represent the same relatively few interest groups, primarily those of health care producers.   The potential recipients of health care are only nominally involved.   Radical changes are unlikely to occur if for no other reason than, as Fox has observed, those involved in the applied field of public policy have in practice no alternative but to give some degree of acceptance to the status quo and behave '. . . "as if" they accepted pluralist assumptions and values.' (55)

(1)   A.Flanders, Management and Unions: The Theory and Reform of
Industrial Relations, Faber, London 1970, p.114.

(2)   Royal Commission on the National Health Service, Report, (Merrison
Report), Cmnd. 7615, HMSO, London 1979, para.21.40.

(3)   A.Maynard and A.Walker, Doctor Manpower 1975-2000: Alternative
Forecasts and their Resource Implications, Royal Commission on the NHS,
Research Paper no.4, HMSO, London 1978, p.25.

(4)   Merrison Report, for instance, Table 3.2.

(5)   Committee to Consider the Future Numbers of Medical Practitioners
and the Appropriate Intake of Medical Students, Report, (Willink
Report), HMSO, London 1957.

(6)   Joint Working Party on the Medical Staffing Structure in the
Hospital Service, Report, (Platt Report), HMSO, London 1961.

(7)   E.Shore, 'Medical Manpower Planning', Health Trends, vol.6, no.2,
May 1974, p.34.

(8)   R.E.Klein, 'Policy Options for Medical Manpower', British Medical
Journal, 9 July 1977.

(9)   Merrison Report, para.14.15.

(10)   Ministry of Health and Ministry of Labour and National Service,
Staffing the Hospitals - An Urgent National Need, HMSO, London 1945.

(11)   A.F.Long and G.Mercer, 'Nurses Down the Drain', Nursing Mirror,
23 November 1978.

(12)   Committee of Enquiry into the Pay and Related Conditions of
Service of the Professions Supplementary to Medicine and Speech
Therapists, Report, (Halsbury Report), HMSO, London 1975.

(13)   Council for Professions Supplementary to Medicine, Annual Report
1977/78, London 1978, p.11;   and M.Blunt, 'Planning the Paramedics: The
Case of Occupational Therapy', Chapter Three of this volume.

(14)   B.L.Donald, 'Towards a More Positive Manpower Policy', Health
Services Manpower Review, vol.3, no.3, August 1977.

(15)   N.Parry and J.Parry, The Rise of the Medical Profession, Croom
Helm, London 1976.

(16)   Klein, 'Policy Options for Medical Manpower'.

(17)   It should be made clear at this point that it is no part of the
objectives of this chapter to argue that restrictive activities by
professions are all that prevent 'rational' manpower planning;   the
intention is merely to show different versions of rationality.   It is
probable that NHS professions as a whole have been less restrictive than
they might have been.   See Merrison Report, para.15.6.

(18)   Reference has already been made to the uneven distribution of
health manpower.   There is no particular reason to assume that
unemployment among health workers would correct rigidities of this kind.
The coexistence of chronic labour shortages in the south east of England
with structural unemployment in the north east suggests that it would
not.   It may be recalled that in 1976, at the height of fears about
overproduction of nurses, it was often argued that there were sufficient
vacancies but not in the areas where nurses were being trained.

(19)   M.J.Nelson, 'Labour Market Survey', Health Services Manpower
Review, vol.2, no.2, May 1976, gives an example of the continuation of a
major capital project in the face of estimations of severe recruitment
difficulty.

(20)   'NHS Planning: The Use of Staffing Norms and Indicators for
Manpower Planning', DHSS letter from C.P.Goodale to Regional and Area
administrators, April 1978.   This contains a bibliography for the bulk

of such norms. The DHSS series of Guides to Good Practice are examples of norms based on work study, whilst patient dependency is the basis of the 'Aberdeen' formula for nurse staffing.

(21) This is now widely recognised: see, for instance, R.Hyman and I.Brough, Social Values and Industrial Relations, Blackwell, Oxford 1975, pp.13-15.

(22) A.Scott-Samuel, 'The Politics of Health', Community Medicine, 1, 1979, p.124.

(23) See: DHSS, The NHS Planning System, HC(76)30, Figure 5; Closure or Change of Use of Health Buildings, HSC(IS)207, 1975; Department of Employment, Employment Protection Act 1975, HMSO, London 1975, Ch.71, sections 17-21; Disclosure of Information to Trade Unions for Collective Bargaining Purposes, Code of Practice no.2, HMSO, London 1977; Health and Safety at Work Act 1974, HMSO, London 1974, Ch.37.

(24) At the time of writing the Nurses and Midwives Council is committed to such a reduction, whilst efforts by the Professional and Technical 'B' Council Staff Side to achieve a reduction are also in progress.

(25) C.J.Ham, 'Power, Patients and Pluralism', in K.A.Barnard and K.Lee (eds), Conflicts in the National Health Service, Croom Helm, London 1977, p.117.

(26) Maynard and Walker, Doctor Manpower, p.1, makes clear not only that possibilities for substitution of doctors exist, but that these 'may have significant resource implications'.

(27) Committee of Enquiry into the Cost of the National Health Service, Report, (Guillebaud Report), Cmnd. 9663, HMSO, London 1956; Joint Working Party on the Medical Staffing Structure in the Hospital Service, Report, (Platt Report), HMSO, London 1961; Royal Commission on Medical Education, Report, (Todd Report), Cmnd. 3569, HMSO, London 1978.

(28) S.R.Engleman, 'External Economic Influences on NHS Manpower', in G.McLachlan, B.Stocking and R.F.A.Shegog (eds), Patterns for Uncertainty? Planning for the Greater Medical Profession, Nuffield Provincial Hospitals Trust, Oxford University Press, Oxford 1979, p.171.

(29) Empirically, it is difficult to see any consistent correlation between NHS manpower distribution and these factors: see, Merrison Report, Ch.3. For an argument that the relationship between health care resources generally and need is an inverse one, see J.T.Hart, 'The Inverse Care Law', Lancet, 1, 1971, p.405.

(30) It has to be recognised that many service changes are simply the aggregation of day to day decisions by NHS workers. Examples are the numbers of diagnostic tests ordered, or outpatients seen, which are aggregate clinical decisions. This situation is not unique to clinicians however but can occur wherever staff make judgements about the use of resources: for example, ward sisters and the frequency of changes of bed linen.

(31) Long and Mercer, 'Nurses Down the Drain', p.18.

(32) B.L.Donald, Manpower for Hospitals, Institute of Hospital Administrators, London 1966.

(33) Maynard and Walker, Doctor Manpower, p.8.

(34) Parry and Parry, The Rise of the Medical Profession, p.228.

(35) Lord McCarthy, Making Whitley Work, HMSO, London 1976.

(36) Engleman, 'External Economic Influences on NHS Manpower', p.175.

(37) This wastage can be, and often is, quite accurately forecast by planners and educators. This does not mean to say that there is any clear causal relationship between changes in entry policy, for example, a school of nursing's decision to increase entry criteria above the

minimum, and changes in this rate.   Nor should it be forgotten that trainees (especially nurses) can be a source of labour.

(38)   Committee on Nursing, Report, (Briggs Report), Cmnd. 5115, HMSO, London 1972, paras.479, 643, 644.

(39)   B.Stocking, 'Confusion or Control? Manpower in the Complementary Health Professions', in McLachlan et al. (eds), Patterns for Uncertainty?, pp.83-107, gives details of the mechanisms relating to manpower in the non medical health professions.

(40)   DHSS, Staffing of the NHS (England): An Analysis of the Demand and Supply Positions in the Major Staff Groups, DHSS, London 1976, para.2.8.

(41)   Parry and Parry, The Rise of the Medical Profession, p.229.

(42)   Shore, 'Medical Manpower Planning', p.33.

(43)   DHSS, Medical Manpower - The Next Twenty Years, HMSO, London 1978, para.100.

(44)   Thus, inability to obtain a consultant in, say, mental handicap would endanger the whole provision of inpatient services for that care group.   Inability to recruit a physiotherapist might endanger a day hospital development.

(45)   B.Crick, In Defence of Politics, Pelican, Harmondsworth 1964, p.21.

(46)   Ibid., p.109.

(47)   K.Ray, 'Manpower Planning - A Systematic Approach', Local Government Chronicle, 24 June 1977, p.519.

(48)   Donald, 'Towards a More Positive Manpower Policy', p.19.

(49)   D.H.Gray, Manpower Planning, Institute of Personnel Management, London 1976, p.16.

(50)   T.L.Hall and M.Kleczkowski, 'Manpower Planning and the Political Process', in T.L.Hall and A.Mejia (eds), Health Manpower Planning, World Health Organisation, Geneva 1978, p.299.

(51)   Ibid., p.303.

(52)   D.Keeling, Management in Government, Allen and Unwin, London 1972, p.108.

(53)   See for instance: Donald, 'Towards a More Positive Manpower Policy', p.25; and Stocking, 'Confusion or Control?', p.104.   The Royal Commission was unable to accept the suggestion, Merrison Report, para.12.62.

(54)   Gray, Manpower Planning, p.12.

(55)   A.Fox, 'Industrial Relations: A Social Critique of Pluralist Ideology', in J.Child (ed.), Man and Organisation, Allen and Unwin, London 1973, p.230.

6 The Role of the DHSS
R. Petch

It might be thought that the need for effective NHS manpower planning
would be self-evident.   So it would seem if one analysed the nature of
health care and the organisation required to deliver it on a
nationalised basis.   Health care is provided by a mix of people -
ranging from the very highly skilled professional to the general manual
labourer - working together at appropriate times and places.   About
60 per cent of the workforce comes from the health professions, in
respect of which the state is both the financial provider of training
and by far the largest source of employment.   Manpower accounts for
75 per cent of revenue expenditure.   Prudent government requires
therefore both that the numbers of people entering such training should
be controlled with as carefully judged regard to future likely
affordable need (hereinafter referred to as demand) as possible and that
the recipients of that training should subsequently so far as possible
be effectively deployed.   The requirements of enlightened personnel
management - and of trade unions - moreover demand that staff should
have secure employment and reasonable career progression.

These desiderata together indicate that the application of manpower
planning in all its aspects (policies on training, recruitment, pay and
retirement) and in all its dimensions (geographical level and location,
unidisciplinary structure and multidisciplinary deployment) needs to be
at the heart of the NHS management process.   Why has such an integrated
approach to manpower planning taken so long to materialise?

The answer to this question must lie primarily in the virtual absence
of effective health service planning generally until the 1970s.   It is
however also found in the fact that the NHS is not regarded or managed
as a corporate entity (this largely accounts for the inadequate flow of
manpower data to the centre) and in the historically prevailing tendency
for the NHS to be managed in a unidisciplinary, vertical fashion with a
consequent compartmentalisation of activity as between the great variety

Acknowledgement   The author wishes to place on record the invaluable
help in the development of manpower planning at the DHSS of Professor
D.Bartholomew, J.S.Gough and A.R.Smith.   The views expressed here are
his own, based on his experience until December 1979.

of professions and trades represented in the service.

This chapter outlines the attempts made since 1974 by the DHSS - working in close collaboration with Regional Health Authorities - to give practical expression to the general desire and evident need for effective manpower planning. In so doing, the role of the centre in developing manpower planning in the NHS is explored and also the place manpower considerations occupy in policy making. The main lesson to be drawn is that manpower planning must be a continuous process, sensitive to changing circumstances. It cannot be based on the conclusions of bodies set up ad hoc or at infrequent intervals, no matter how well considered these are. (1)

THE NEW WORLD OF 1974

The reorganisation of the NHS and of the DHSS leading up to April 1974 created a structure within which planning in all its aspects could in principle effectively be undertaken. It is indeed arguable that the emerging planning system offered 'the essential means of arranging the de facto reorganisation of the NHS' (2) or, put another way, that 'planning welds the NHS into the kind of organic whole that its creators envisaged and hoped for.' (3)

Manpower planning was seen as an integral feature of the new personnel function, which *inter alia* was established in order to 'ensure that all groups of staff have the benefit of the advice, support and procedures provided by specialist personnel staff, and that to the maximum possible extent common policies and procedures apply to all.' (4) Within DHSS, a branch (P4C) was created to promote the development of the NHS personnel function. Like the function itself, this branch was by no means plentifully resourced by comparison with other large national organisations; and in the early days the main effort had perforce to be devoted to establishments work and the problems associated with a changing industrial relations climate and a welter of new employment legislation. There was moreover as yet no overall planning framework within which manpower planning could take its place.

This strategy led to the promotion between 1977 and 1979 of three initiatives which together have enabled an integrated approach to manpower planning to be developed. The first was the reconstitution in the autumn of 1976 of the Joint Manpower Planning and Information Working Group (MAPLIN) in a form which facilitated a continuing dialogue between DHSS and manpower planners at Regional level. The second was the creation in the summer of 1978 of the Manpower Intelligence Branch (MIB) within DHSS. The third was the extension of the DHSS planning system to the NHS, and in particular the 1978-79 round of strategic plans within which health authorities were specifically asked to give manpower considerations their due weight.

Prior to its reconstruction in 1976, MAPLIN had filled the limited but necessary role of providing a forum in which a standardised approach to the collection, storing and dissemination of manpower data could be hammered out between DHSS and the representatives of the NHS. (5) In its reconstituted role, however, MAPLIN was charged with the greater responsibilities of developing manpower planning expertise within the NHS and ensuring that the skills of manpower planners were properly recognised. The membership of MAPLIN was of crucial importance for this purpose. Each of the 14 RHAs in England was asked to nominate a member of its staff to become the 'focal point' for manpower planning within the Region, thus ensuring both national coverage and a specified status for the focal points. In the event, 13 RHAs nominated a member of the personnel department and the other a computer services officer with close connections with his personnel department. The new MAPLIN also included a 'Composite Regional Team of Officers' (an Administrator, Medical Officer, Nursing Officer, Treasurer and Works Officer) and a Regional Personnel Officer. This was to ensure that there was a member of each main Regional discipline sufficiently involved with the development of NHS manpower planning to represent the manpower planning interest at meetings of his or her discipline. The new MAPLIN membership also included NHS manpower planners from Scotland and Wales, and representatives from the English, Welsh and Scottish Health Departments.

MAPLIN discussions have veered between the broad strategic and the detailed technical. In order to accommodate such diverse interests, MAPLIN occasions have sometimes more resembled public meetings than working group discussions. To overcome this, MAPLIN has assumed a more federal structure. The Regional officers together with senior officers from DHSS form a steering group. The focal points and their DHSS counterparts meet as a forum for the exchange of information and ideas - that is, as a technical group.

The MIB was established in 1978 to perform the 'DHSS Manpower Intelligence Function for the NHS'. It was formed by bringing together the administrative staff responsible for sponsoring the development of the NHS personnel function (these staff had been known as the Manpower Intelligence Unit since October 1976) and the statisticians and their support staff with related responsibilities for NHS manpower statistics. A manpower planner was also seconded from the NHS. At the same time a number of other staff who were already engaged in manpower planning work were designated as part-time members of MIB. This built into the MIB a wide range of professional and technical expertise. The part-time members included staff from the Economic Adviser's Office, from Operational Research Services, from Management Services and Computers Divisions together with representatives of Medical and Nursing Divisions. Additionally, close links were established with the administrative branches responsible for the personnel management of individual NHS staff groups (especially doctors and nurses) and with the branches responsible for the development of service policies.

In 1976 a comprehensive corporate planning system was introduced to the NHS. The framework it provided to match, among other things, manpower with service provision has already been outlined in Chapter Two. The first round of strategic planning in 1976-77 took little specific account of manpower. For the second round in 1978-79, health authorities were asked 'to quantify so far as possible the manpower implications of their service plans and in particular to estimate, by broad staff group, their likely manpower requirements in 1981 and 1988.' (6) In addition, a number of long term manpower supply assumptions were made available to assist Authorities in this task.

103

The great importance of the 1978-79 planning round in relation to manpower planning is that in principle it should for the first time provide a set of estimates of forward demand for NHS manpower based on detailed service planning. It is difficult to predict how useful these demand estimates will be; but the fact that they will have been compiled at all will mark a major step forward in NHS manpower planning. MIB is examining these strategic plans with especial regard to the staffing levels and mixes implied by the plans, the consistency between financial, service and manpower projections, and the extent to which known supply constraints have been allowed for. As a result of this process, various discussions will take place with a view *inter alia* to enabling more satisfactory manpower demand projections to be made in the next round of strategic planning.

DHSS ROLE AND ACHIEVEMENTS

As was meiotically stated in 1978, 'the Department recognises that manpower planning is a complex process and that it will take some time to develop it fully.' (7)   What then is the role of the centre in manpower planning?   In brief, MIB's task is to collect relevant information and to present it in such forms as will assist decision makers.   It is not itself charged with making decisions about such matters as manpower recruitment, training and deployment.   It exists to ensure that such decisions will be progressively better informed.   The remainder of this chapter explores in greater detail the various aspects of the DHSS manpower intelligence function.

Roles and relationships

With the creation of MIB, the DHSS has succeeded in brigading the several components concerned with manpower intelligence to increase its effectiveness.   Efforts are concentrated in four areas.   Firstly, it tries to monitor the deployment of NHS manpower.   This mainly involves compiling, maintaining and using sufficiently comprehensive data on NHS employees.   One of the first requests made to DHSS by the Royal Commission on the NHS was for information about the current and likely future NHS workforce.   The resultant document is regarded as an extremely useful synoptic account of NHS manpower at national level and was widely distributed. (8)   It is now subject to periodic updating.

Secondly, MIB attempts to ensure that at national level, quantitative manpower implications are brought to bear upon policy formulation, personnel and operational management, strategic planning, and research and development.   This involves regular and frequent liaison with all parts of the health side of DHSS as well as such bodies as the National Staff Committees.   The MIB has thus developed an extensive network of contacts within DHSS aimed at ensuring that manpower considerations play their rightful part in the generation of policies of all kinds.

Thirdly, MIB is concerned with encouraging within each Region the establishment of an appropriate manpower planning capability and the dissemination of adequate manpower intelligence.   This involves co-ordinating Regional Health Authorities towards a common and consistent approach to manpower planning.   The activities of MAPLIN have undoubtedly led to the progressive development of a manpower planning capability within each RHA, and of a forum within which manpower intelligence can be exchanged. (9)

Finally, under this heading, MIB has an overall aim of ensuring that line managers throughout the NHS are sufficiently aware of the relevance of manpower planning to their management role. This involves arranging that manpower planning is adequately covered in all forms of management training. MIB has assisted a number of Regions to arrange manpower planning training events for NHS managers. (10)

Data base

The *sine qua non* of any respectable manpower planning is an adequate base of data about manpower stocks and flows. Such a base has never existed in the NHS. It is not infrequently argued that until such time as significant improvements have been made in this field manpower planning might just as well not be attempted. There is no reason in principle why this sad state of affairs should exist: as the Royal Commission pointed out, the required data 'should be available locally.' (11)

The problem lies in getting the data through the various levels of the NHS and to DHSS in a form that each level can use for the performance of its function. This depends more than anything else upon establishing a mutually satisfactory system of occupational coding. Despite various initiatives in the past, this has never been achieved. A MAPLIN working party is currently examining the problem in depth as a matter of urgency.

For the generality of NHS staff, the national manpower information system was developed largely for wage bargaining purposes. It comprises in essence a simple headcount conducted annually on 30 September by employing Authorities (that is, broad geographical location), staff group and grade, sex, and whole-time equivalents as well as actual numbers. In relation to wage bargaining itself, the system allows little more sophistication than the mere costing of pay settlements. It does not permit of the kind of approach indicated (but not adopted) by the Clegg Commission when it said recently that 'labour supply is clearly relevant to pay determination.' (12) This also underlines the need for better NHS manpower intelligence generally. (13)

The seriousness of these deficiencies is accepted within DHSS. MIB is therefore concerned with promoting standardisation of terminology and occupational coding, to allow aggregated and valid comparisons on NHS manpower to be made. It also seeks to ensure that the regular collection at the appropriate level of adequate statistical information about NHS personnel, covering both analyses of stocks and measurement of flows. Finally, it aims to maintain at national level a data base showing quantitative and qualitative characteristics of staff in post by reference to staff group, geographical location (down to at least Regional level), and health programme. This is necessary for management purposes in order to answer such a question as 'How many and what kind of nurses are employed in the Northern Region on the care of the elderly?'. The degree of detail in which the data are maintained varies between staff groups and must have regard primarily to the perceived needs of management at different levels in the NHS.

A long term solution has been sought in agreeing to sponsor the
development of a Standard Manpower Planning and Personnel Information
System (STAMP) to complement the Standard Accounting System and the
Standard Payroll System. STAMP is being developed by Wessex Regional
Health Authority as a Centre of Responsibility, and its features and
role are discussed in Chapter Four of this book. The development of
STAMP, and of the common format of data which it implies, of course
depends primarily upon co-operation between all levels of the NHS
(including DHSS). MAPLIN provides an ideal forum for this co-operation
to be achieved.

But STAMP will not of itself necessarily assist the development of
more reliable demand forecasting. If as expected the planning system
is to continue to be based on a care group disaggregation, more work
will be needed to refine the allocation of staff to care groups. The
development of clinical budgeting and speciality costing will facilitate
this refinement. Certain staff groups such as administrative and
clerical staff cannot readily be allocated to one care group or
another; and other staff groups (for example, community nurses) divide
their time between patients in different care groups. Agreed
conventions will be needed before these problems can be tackled.

Supply forecasting

The inadequacies of the existing data base have greatly hampered the
development of supply forecasting for NHS staff. It is desirable that
supply forecasting should be undertaken at the level appropriate to the
type of labour market from which staff are drawn; and DHSS activity in
this area should therefore in principle be confined to those whose
labour market is national or international.

The clearest case is that of doctors. Here, the DHSS Operational
Research Services (ORS) have developed a model which is described in the
consultative document *Medical Manpower - The Next Twenty Years*. (14)
The model is designed to demonstrate the long term effects of changes in
medical school intake on the national stock of doctors inside and outside the NHS. Other medical manpower models are being developed. So
far as the supply of doctors in individual specialities is concerned,
DHSS issues annual guidelines to Regions about the supply of fully-
trained doctors. These now include estimates of the numbers of
additional consultant posts which are likely to be approved in the
shortage specialities in the following financial year. The Department
also publishes an article every year in *Health Trends* about the recruitment position in the different specialities; this is intended to act as
a basis for careers advice to young doctors.

ORS have also developed a supply model for nurses. This has two main
functions. One is to enable the future nursing labour force to be
estimated on the basis of a range of options for the size of entry into
nurse training. The other - its converse - is to estimate the desired
size of entry into nurse training on the basis of different estimates of
future demand. This model is capable of substantial development as
data improve. Attempts are currently being made to adapt it to
simulate both particular specialisms within the national nurse manpower
system and the sub-national nursing systems at Regional level. The
latter will be particularly important if individual Regions are to

become self-sufficient in nurse training.

For other staff groups, attempts have been made to use the MANPLAN computer models developed by the Civil Service Department. One such exercise was carried out for the National Staff Committee concerned with the National Administrative Trainee Scheme. This enabled the Committee to take a better-informed decision about the desirable entry into this scheme. (15) There is considerable scope for this kind of activity at national level in respect of the professions supplementary to medicine and some of the scientific and technical groups. But as already indicated, this work is substantially inhibited by deficiencies in the national data base.

In this area, MIB is therefore concerned to obtain agreement on the lowest management level at which supply forecasting for any staff group should take place and ensure that it is adequately undertaken at that level, and as necessary by aggregation at higher levels. The determination depends upon the size of the relevant labour market, ranging from international for doctors and dentists through to local for ancillary staff. The execution depends on adequate liaison with other agencies concerned, both within and without the NHS, and - where it needs to be undertaken at national level (notably in respect of doctors) - requires the maintenance of a data base with respect to overall potential supply. In essence then, MIB aims to ensure that supply considerations are brought to bear upon all aspects of management, especially in relation to policy formulation, personnel management and capital developments. Through MAPLIN, assistance is provided to Regional Health Authorities, and through them Area Health Authorities, to develop techniques for forecasting local labour supply, where appropriate.

Demand forecasting

If manpower supply forecasting is relatively underdeveloped in the NHS, *a fortiori* is this the case in respect of demand forecasting. One of the reasons for this is that, unlike supply forecasting, its demand counterpart can in general only be sensibly undertaken horizontally (that is, across all staff groups) on account of the multidisciplinary nature of the provision of health care.

Part of the MIB role here must be to estimate the future national demand for health manpower implied by current and proposed national policies. As indicated earlier, one of the first requests made by the Royal Commission on the NHS to the DHSS was for an estimate of the likely NHS workforce in ten years' time. The resultant figures were compiled by the DHSS Economic Adviser's Office on the basis of forward financial projections, taking into account historical trends in the growth rates of the main staff groups relative to the growth of revenue in volume terms. (16) Since financial projections are undertaken in terms of service provision, it is possible to build up manpower forecasts on a similar basis. This global approach is clearly insensitive to likely changes in operational activities. The manpower forecasts thus obtained can be no more than rough guides to the future. Nonetheless, this approach is capable of being applied at Regional and local level and has been commended through MAPLIN accordingly.

Much more satisfactory would be a compilation of manpower demand forecasts on the basis of local service planning. As already stated, the
1978-79 round of NHS strategic planning provided the first opportunity
for this to be undertaken. The problems in so doing were however
considerable. On the one hand, there was a lack of manpower data
collected on the basis of the type of health care on which staff are
engaged. On the other, there was a general lack of agreed criteria
upon which staffing needs for any given level of service could be
assessed. On this latter point, it was agreed to gather together all
the extant guidance on staffing levels issued over time, preceding this
with an introduction analysing the various types of 'staffing norm' with
some indication of the pitfalls accompanying each. The resultant
letter to Regional and Area Administrators was probably the most useful
single document issued by MIB to date. (17)

But health authorities were left to their own devices in respect of
the numerous areas of health care provision for which no staffing
standards existed. The present (and foreseeable) economic climate is
inhospitable to the development of further staffing norms, which tend to
connote ideal standards on the basis of the best current practice.
What can the DHSS do in these circumstances to assist health authorities
to develop credible methods of demand forecasting?

The best approach seems to be that of gaining more knowledge as to how
NHS manpower is currently utilised. If the actual deployment of NHS
manpower at all levels can be more satisfactorily mapped out, it should
become progressively more possible for judgements to be made - again, at
the appropriate level - as to the directions in which change should be
planned. One method of applying this approach already referred to is
the attempt to relate staffing statistics to the kind of health care
activity upon which staff are engaged. Another is for DHSS to provide
feedback of aggregated staffing statistics in such a way that health
authorities can relate their own staff utilisation to that elsewhere, by
reference to such measures as catchment population, patient throughput,
and other staff groups.

Another potentially helpful approach in guiding health authorities
towards more satisfactory demand forecasting is the dissemination of
'good staffing practice' on the basis of management services and
research studies. (18)   Again, MAPLIN provides a suitable forum for
this.   Yet another is the development of regression analysis techniques
for analysis of the historic path that has led to existing staffing
patterns; and this too is being attempted in some locations with the
active help of the DHSS.

Matching supply and demand

As is evident from the previous sections of this chapter, much work
needs to be done on manpower information, and forecasting both supply
and demand.   Only then will the matching of supply and demand have any
real credibility. . A critical part of MIB's role must therefore be to
try to ensure that any substantial foreseeable mismatches between
estimated supply and demand, after due allowance for the inevitable
uncertainties, are brought to the attention of management so that
appropriate action may be taken in good time.   Corrective policies
could involve supply (recruitment, training, pay) and/or demand (health

care priorities, technology, professional roles) and might involve the
negotiation of desirable options which would not emerge without the
evidence of need provided by the manpower intelligence.

So far DHSS has unfortunately only been able to provide limited
assistance in this area.   Often it was compelled to fall back on some
generalisation such as 'nursing manpower overall is expected to increase
slowly at about the rate of general growth, though within nursing the
demand for particular groups is likely to be much stronger . . .' (19)
The comparable section in the following year's planning guidelines
assuredly indicates a considerable advance. (20)   The MIB is now being
asked for help increasingly, indicating that it is succeeding in its aim
of raising manpower consciousness in general.   The prime need is to
improve the quality of assistance.

Manpower control and utilisation

The final aspect of the manpower intelligence function is to ensure that
those concerned with manpower control and utilisation are supplied with
comparative data about the deployment and utilisation of NHS manpower.
This essentially involves undertaking management-oriented analyses of
the statistical data base.   Current and foreseeable financial
stringency renders it especially essential that NHS manpower should be
deployed with the maximum possible efficiency and effectiveness.   The
extent to which this is so can only be revealed by the assiduous
comparison of manpower statistics over time, between geographical level,
and by activity.

CONCLUSION

The purpose of this chapter has been to indicate current perceptions
about the DHSS role in manpower planning in the NHS.   The role agreed
for the manpower intelligence function at DHSS is indeed a large one,
encompassing demand forecasting, influences over supply (through
training and pay), fostering research and new developments (such as
STAMP), and stimulating and encouraging manpower planning in the health
service (particularly through the workings of MAPLIN).

One might easily conclude that it is all very well in theory but quite
impossible to put into practice.   Manpower planning for the NHS is
indeed a protean activity.   A fundamental concern is to establish a
satisfactory manpower planning capability within the NHS itself.   As
this is progressively achieved, it should be possible for the DHSS to
reduce its own involvement and to concentrate on the areas for which
NHS manpower planning can sensibly be undertaken only at national level.

NOTES

(1) For example, the experience of medical manpower planning - DHSS, Medical Manpower - The Next Twenty Years, HMSO, London 1978, Ch.1.

(2) C.Graham, internal DHSS memo, 13 April 1976.

(3) Mrs.E.Körner, 'The Importance of Being Earnest about Planning', Hospital and Health Services Review, October 1979.

(4) DHSS, Operation and Development of Services: Organisation for Personnel Management, NHS Reorganisation Circular HRC(73)37, DHSS, London 1973, para.18.

(5) Testaments to its role are the following MAPLIN Reports: DHSS, Leavers (Standard Measures and Classifications), DHSS, London 1975; DHSS, Absence from Work, DHSS, London 1975.

(6) DHSS, Planning Guidelines for 1978-79, HC(78)12, DHSS, London 1978, Part 6.

(7) Ibid.

(8) DHSS, Staffing of the NHS (England): An Analysis of the Demand and Supply Positions in the Major Staff Groups, DHSS, London 1979, latest edition.

(9) The establishment of NHS Manpower News (from DHSS/MIB, first edition February 1979) and Personnel Information Papers (from NHS Regional Personnel Officers - for example, PIPS, no.7, North Western RHA, October 1979) provide vehicles for the wider dissemination of information on manpower matters.

(10) The manpower information training package outlined in Chapter Four is an example of such a role.

(11) Royal Commission on the National Health Service, Report, (Merrison Report), Cmnd. 7615, HMSO, London 1979, para.12.64.

(12) Standing Commission on Pay Comparability, (Clegg Commission), Report No.1 - Local Authority and University Manual Workers, NHS Ancillary Staffs, and Ambulancemen, HMSO, London 1979, Cmnd. 7641, para.59.

(13) Information on medical and dental manpower is a great deal more comprehensive, as health authorities provide personal and contractual details for each doctor and dentist in their staffing returns. This permits detailed analysis by grade, specialty, age, sex, place of birth, and also provides a basis for deriving information about movements.

(14) DHSS, Medical Manpower, Appendix C.

(15) National Staff Committee for Administrative and Clerical Staff, The Recruitment and Career Development of Administrators, DHSS, London 1978.

(16) DHSS, Staffing of the NHS, paras.1.4 to 1.9.

(17) 'NHS Planning: The Use of Staffing Norms and Indicators for Manpower Planning', DHSS letter from C.P.Goodale to Regional and Area administrators, April 1978.

(18) D.Lewin, 'An Approach to Area Strategic Planning: Report for the Operational Research Service of the DHSS', unpublished report, February 1979.

(19) DHSS, Planning Guidelines for 1978-79, Part 6, para.6.8.

(20) DHSS, Planning Guidelines for 1979-80, HC(79)9, DHSS, London 1979, Part 4, paras.4.14 to 4.21.

7 Manpower in Strategic Planning at the Regional Level

REGIONAL PRACTICE: THE FOCAL POINT VIEW

A.F. Long and *G. Mercer*

Manpower planning within the NHS received a new urgency following the introduction of the corporate planning system in 1976. The Region's role in this context is to develop a strategic plan covering a 10 year period, and to assess and monitor strategic and operational plans from Areas and Districts. The first steps produced in the 1976 round indicated that most plans contained little or no consideration of manpower implications. This raised doubts about the manpower planning capability within the NHS which must be of a higher standard to justify further devolution of responsibilities.

How the Region should interpret and implement its strategic function is not predetermined. It could see its place as being to draw up guidelines for Areas covering such issues as preferred service objectives, norms for manpower and service provision, and the format of the service plan. Areas' strategic plans would then be assessed for their correspondence to such guidelines. The resultant Regional plan would comprise a summation of these Area strategies, modified where appropriate. That describes what is known as the 'bottom up' approach. It contrasts with the more directive and independent role which a Region could play. In this guise the Region would formulate the corporate objectives and draw up the strategy itself. Consultation would follow with Areas to organise their contribution to the overall strategy. This is termed the 'top down' approach.

The major part of this chapter comprises two case studies of these contrasting approaches to strategic planning with specific reference to the manpower input in the 1978/79 round. In Blunt's discussion of the practice in Trent RHA the bottom up perspective is emphasised, while Dixon and Cree illustrate the form which the converse approach has assumed in Wessex. Especially in the infancy of the NHS planning system more than one viewpoint is to be expected, if not encouraged. Meaningful evaluation must wait until the plans have been fully implemented and monitored.

A similar testing period in the early years characterises the work of the individual focal points who, from their membership of MAPLIN, are charged with the responsibility for stimulating manpower planning. In order to provide a wider context for the contrasting approaches examined in the Trent and Wessex case studies it is worthwhile commenting briefly on Regional experiences across the country. The material derives from a survey of focal points conducted by the authors. (1)

The novelty of the focal point position and the range of acceptance of manpower planning, and of the manpower component in planning, across and within Regions, has led to significant variations in practice. In general, the focal points' contribution was recognised in their membership of the Regional planning team. In a substantial minority of Regions this did not extend far beyond a formalised involvement. The survey analysis suggested a gulf between those focal points' activities in Regions with real commitment to developing the manpower component in Regional strategic planning, and other RHAs where so little conviction and resources were invested. The risk is that they will play little more than a supernumerary function. Nevertheless, widespread agreement was expressed on their proper role. Primarily it involved co-ordination, both promoting manpower planning, being its enabler, catalyst or innovator, as well as providing manpower information. The necessity of liaising with the broader planning division and medical/dental planners was also evident.

It is actual practice which revealed how differently focal points were expected to promote manpower planning. At one extreme, the focal point's contribution was restricted to providing advice on how to complete the summary manpower table in the SASP forms. At the other end of the spectrum, the focal point was involved in the creation of a complete methodology for the manpower input and for planning overall. The crucial factor is less whether the Region is committed more to a top down rather than a bottom up approach, but more simply whether within the individual Region manpower consciousness is sufficiently advanced to demand informed activity in this field. Specifically, focal points were most regularly contacted for advice on the completion of the SASP table, to help with manpower data and information generally, and to provide norms and guidelines on staff groups. Supply and demand fore-casting of a more sophisticated sort, and assessment of the financial resources required, were infrequently requested. If there was a typical Region, the focal point was attempting to stimulate manpower planning through stressing its need - both at Region and in local health authorities. There would be discussion with interested persons on data requirements and the provision of comparative manpower norms. Little other activity of noteworthy significance would be conducted.

Approaches adopted to generating the demand for manpower within planning indicated the domination of norms, national averages and professional judgement. Specific mention was also made that demands for manpower arose from the summation of Area planning requirements, with the minority proviso that estimates of likely supply and finance had to be taken into account. As often as not focal points were providing information for demand forecasts in response to ad hoc requests rather than to support a systematic 'bottom up' analysis. In only one Region was a model developed which allowed a calculation of future levels of staff against the 1976 outturn for each care group, in a 'top down' format.

On the supply side of the manpower equation there was little variation
reported by focal points. For all Regions consideration of this aspect
was very limited. In some cases analyses were made of the economically
active population now and in 10 years' time in terms of its total size,
or selective labour market surveys were used, or probable shortfalls in
supply noted. Overall, consideration of supply was very limited,
identifying possible supply constraints and not moving on to the
difficult yet essential issue of generating policies which might remedy
the position.

The consideration given to the supply of manpower was echoed in focal
points' perceptions of the potential influence of RHAs on their manpower
supply. The general comment was that there was little or no influence
that could be brought to bear, that it was difficult to judge the
potential influence, or that the whole subject was simply unexplored.
The role of modifying training intake levels in line with recruitment
(and turnover) patterns was one presumed tactic. Which tier could
exercise most influence depended on the staff group. The general
conclusion can only be that the possibility of exerting a noteworthy
impact on supply was as yet disregarded or not investigated. In
practice authorities tended to focus on the nursing and midwifery staff,
which reflects not only the size and contribution that this group makes
to the NHS but also to the comparatively greater acceptance among senior
nursing staff of the need for manpower planning.

The most common difficulty in developing the manpower input to the
1978/79 round of strategic planning was expressed as an inadequate
information base. Problems were reported because it was restricted in
scope, it lacked accuracy, and was often difficult to access. There
was also a need for an information base that dovetailed with the
planner's concept of a care group. Yet other shortcomings in current
practice were perceived in the estimation of demand, either through
lacking manpower norms or through an absence of confidence in making
subjective judgements within manpower forecasts. The problems raised
led to suggestions that planning guidelines should contain indications
of likely manpower problems. Recruitment difficulties should be
explored and worked through to the consequences of future supply and
back to manpower demands, and in this way modify the service plans.
Finally, the thorny issue of supply forecasting, and what influence NHS
authorities might exert, had to be tackled.

Not only were there doubts about the technical basis of manpower
planning in health authorities but consternation was often expressed
about the general lack of support for such activities. There was
frequent mention that the lines of responsibility were too faintly
drawn. Respondents reported poor acceptance or lack of awareness of
the manpower aspects of plans, both by planners and personnel officers.
Indeed the latter's function in the whole process was typically regarded
as problematic. These comments highlight what the focal points
perceived as the need for a more structured approach to the manpower
input within the Regional level. Chief officers were expected to adopt
a more sympathetic attitude to the manpower contribution to planning,
facilitating links between planners, personnel officers and managers.
In other words, manpower planning had to become an integral part of the

planning process.   This also entailed a closer involvement of the Areas and Districts.

To sum up, focal points emphasised official wisdom on manpower planning as a battery of technical tasks and skills, as well as how the manpower component should fit in with strategic planning.   On balance, focal points agreed with the devolution of manpower planning respons- ibilities to the Region from DHSS, although they were less united or clear about the division among the NHS levels.   At this stage, *force majeure*, the horizon of most focal points was restricted to stimulating manpower consciousness throughout the relevant authorities.   Regional strategic planning is playing its part in pushing the NHS towards a consideration of the manpower component in planning, but evidence of the benefits of good practice in this field are sorely needed to convince the doubters.   The case studies of Trent and Wessex which follow are offered as contrasting perspectives on the Regional contribution, and of possible ways forward despite their admitted tentative and exploratory nature.

A CASE STUDY OF TRENT RHA

M.Blunt

Introduction

Since the inception of the NHS Trent has been the Region most clearly
deprived of health service resources. (2)   Constantly at the bottom of
the national 'league table' in terms of revenue per head of population,
hospitals, equipment and staff, this has resulted in service omissions
to the Region's population.   Through national policies intended to redistribute revenue resources, Trent has grown over the past few years,
and will grow in the coming decade, at a rapid rate towards parity with
national levels of expenditure per head of population.   As much of this
growth requires large numbers of additional staff the planning of
manpower is of major importance.

A major consideration in planning such a growth in staff numbers has
been to break out of the historical 'circle of deprivation' existing in
the Region.   Trent as a 'deprived' Region is unattractive to potential
staff for reasons ranging from lack of physical facilities, equipment
and other staff to the lack of a suitable environment in which to make
a home.   As such, recruitment is difficult and the resulting shortage
of staff only serves to make the Region more unattractive.   Trent,
perhaps more than most Regions, is therefore concerned to plan
effectively the supply and utilisation of its staff.   In turn these
factors can only be planned in response to a clearly defined and
quantified statement of the future demand for staff.   It is primarily
for this reason that manpower planning has become an integral part of
the development of the strategic planning system in Trent.

Background to planning in Trent

The first strategic planning round in 1976 caught the NHS on the
rebound from reorganisation.   In Trent this meant that little was
accomplished to add to late and poor national guidelines for strategic
planning.   Areas were in no real state so soon after their inception to
undertake such a process and thus Area plans were not much more than
broad statements of objectives.   The Regional plan, dependent on Area
plans for its data, could only fall back on previously stated Regional
policy objectives which did not attempt to quantify or fully take into
account resource constraints.   The manpower element of the plan had
nothing to fall back on.   As far as could be ascertained there had
never previously been an attempt to quantify the demand for manpower in
a comprehensive and strategic sense.   The manpower plan was thus
confined to a short analysis of present deprivation against the national
standards.   This consisted of a statement of objectives on the major
staff groups primarily constructed from national standards projected 10
years ahead on broad national and Regional resource assumptions.

Although praised against others' efforts, the plan was by no means
what the Region expected from the planning system.   The period from
1977 to 1978 was one of internal development to improve on the 1976
experience.   The role of the Region's officer service planning team was
defined, and began to function.   Regional and Area level planners began
to recognise their roles and co-ordinate their functions across and

within administrative discipline boundaries. Communication on planning matters measurably improved. Regional authority members and top officers were seen to be taking the planning system seriously. Indeed a Regional authority member steering group and officer working group were formed from Areas and the Region to study and resolve planning system issues. This has resulted in communication, understanding, education and agreement on many facets of both strategic and operational planning.

During 1978 there emerged a clearer understanding of what was required; it remained to be seen whether this understanding could be accomplished in the next round of strategic plans in 1978/79. The Regional service planning team determined three broad major objectives in the construction of plans for 1978/79. Firstly, service plans should be constructed so as to be mindful of resource constraints and to integrate the different resource plans for finance, capital and manpower as much as possible. Secondly, planning should be generally bottom up, that is, generated at local level in order to ensure the best possible statement of future service developments. Thirdly, an attempt should be made in the eventual strategic plan to show what it would seek to do on the resources available to it, and what it would like to do but could not achieve due to resource constraints.

The DHSS in commenting on the 1976 round of Regional plans (3) had stressed the inadequacy of the manpower elements. The Region was therefore concerned to rectify this shortcoming. To arrive at an adequate manpower strategic plan several questions had to be asked of Area plans. Are levels of staffing over or under estimated in the light of likely resource constraints? Are the priorities given to the expansion of different groups of staff correct? Are estimates of staff required likely to be available for employment and if not are there proposals to improve availability? Does the proposed expansion in staff conform with national and Regional guidance? Will the proposed expansion meet the perceived needs for development of services in the Area concerned? In order to ensure, as much as possible, that Area plans gave the Region data which would answer these questions a policy of assisting Areas to construct their manpower plans was evolved.

Manpower methodology

The basic methodology adopted for the manpower element of the strategic planning process arose out of the need to provide policy guidance on manpower development to Areas on which they could base their strategic plans. Such a process should involve the NHS at Regional level in interpreting national guidance in the light of particular Regional needs. However, the national guidance produced was inadequate for this purpose and Regional planners were left in the position of trying to assist and direct Areas in their planning through guidance almost entirely produced at Regional level.

In terms of manpower planning this meant producing guidance in the absence of a Regional baseline of manpower planning policy. However, some major points were identified. By 1988 the Region would in terms of financial resources be much nearer the national standard, and Trent could seek staffing levels consistent with future national levels. As Trent grew towards the levels of expenditure enjoyed by other Regions it could be presumed that the way in which this money was spent on staff would also match that prevailing nationally. This would mean major changes in the mix of staff in Trent. Although the Region had the lowest staffing levels in the country for virtually all of the main groups of staff, this fact masked other and greater relative deprivations of staff. This was brought about by circles of deprivation affecting staff groups who form a larger than Regional labour market (for example, medical and professional and technical staff) rather more than those groups of staff who could be recruited at the District level (for example, nursing and ancillary staff). This meant that Trent had grown in staffing terms in a lop sided fashion in the past, recruiting those staff they could. Thus expenditure on the different staff groups varied considerably from the national pattern of expenditure and similarly varied within the Region due to differing levels of deprivation in different Areas and Districts.

Trent could not immediately follow the national policy emphasising the development of geriatric and mental illness and handicap services. This was due to capital programme commitments to improve the standard of acute accommodation in the Region. The emphasis in staff development during the first five years of the plan would therefore be among those professions particularly concerned with acute care. Although nationally maternity staffing was expected to contract due to falling birth rates Trent, with similarly falling birth rates, still needed to expand maternity staffing to achieve acceptable staffing levels.

Further guidance set out overall targets and constraints for medical, dental and nursing staff in different specialties and likely growth rates for other groups of staff, as well as pointing towards education and training priorities. (4) Any real guidance on potential levels of supply of staff was lacking due to the lack of a comprehensive manpower policy in the Region. The 'chicken and egg' situation of being unable to plan without guidelines and being unable to produce guidelines due to a lack of planning (or policy) severely restricted what could be attempted in the manpower element of the plan. Manpower planners therefore set themselves certain objectives which they thought should be attainable in this round of planning.

As service planning was developing in the form of planning individual health care services, that is a 'programme' type approach to planning, manpower planning would, where possible, attempt to integrate with this approach and produce manpower demand and supply forecasts on a service by service basis. This approach has many difficulties as traditionally manpower information has been collected in a geographic or a service form. Although planners know how many staff worked in a particular hospital they could not easily identify how many of them worked in geriatrics, mental illness, children's services, and so on. This was particularly true of those large groups of staff who provide a servicing function rather than a direct patient care function. These included the professional and technical, ancillary, and administrative and clerical staffs. Yet even with medical and nursing staff such a categorisation was often difficult if not impossible with present data sources. It was therefore recognised at an early stage that the inability to compare proposed service developments with the manpower needed to accomplish them would be a major inadequacy in the 1978/9 strategic planning round.

117

A major drawback in the previous planning round was the inability to study manpower demand against financial constraints. Without study of this fundamental constraint to a development manpower plans could be little more than statements of possibly unattainable objectives. Improvement in the liaison between manpower and financial planning was therefore agreed to be a necessity. In addition, little information existed on the potential supply of staff or how and to what extent this supply could be affected to meet the future demands for staff. It was agreed that, although the attempts to quantify future supply would be very basic, this should be attempted. Without it a real manpower strategy was impossible to formulate.

The Region in its guidance also set standards of conformity for Area plans. They had to adhere to the standard structure for strategic plans as set out in the NHS planning system manual. (5) This would ensure that Areas prepared their plans in a standard form taking into account the major factors and services required by a comprehensive strategic planning process. Secondly, Areas had to complete a set of the Summary Analysis of Strategic Plan (SASP) forms promulgated from national level (and as amended for their manpower elements within the Region). This would ensure, unlike the 1976 plan, that strategies on resources and services could be quantified and assessed. The return of manpower SASP forms especially would allow a Regional consideration of each group and profession of staff as well as analysis of certain professions by health care group thus satisfying the need, at least for medical and nursing staff, to adopt a programme approach to planning. Overall, the demand for conformity further pressured Areas to commit management capacity to the planning round, which reinforced the importance of the system and in turn resulted in the production of better strategies than those produced in 1976.

As the Region could only seek to plan manpower based on locally quantified demands, and Areas lacked expertise and capacity to plan manpower, a major role of the Regional manpower planning section had to be to act as a catalyst, adviser, and assistant to Areas on demand. Some Areas used this facility more than others, and some to greater eventual effect than others. In many ways this involvement opened better channels of communication and trust between Regional and Area manpower planners which are still being consolidated. Areas were visited at their request to discuss with their planning teams or individual officers the Region's requirements, hopes and aspirations for the planning round. The Regional planning guidelines were explained in detail as to how they affected the Area. Ways and means of undertaking the manpower element of the Area plan were also discussed, pointing out systems of information and analysis that may be of use and offering the assistance of the Regional manpower planning section where possible.

Such visits reinforced the view that, of all the elements of planning, Areas were most unsure, most sceptical, and most lacking in their capacity to fulfil the manpower element. Out of this realisation came the idea to feed Areas with information and analyses which had been developed at Region. These analyses were originally constructed in order to give the Region a monitoring tool against which Area plans could be assessed. As such they set parameters within which it was hoped the Areas' manpower strategies would fall. In publishing these analyses as a 'Preliminary Analysis of the Manpower Situation' the

Region was showing the range within which it was expected that the
manpower strategies would fall prior to the receipt of Area plans and,
indeed, prior to the construction of Area strategies. The Regional
manpower planners were, in a sense, publishing unofficial and rough
guesses about what were believed to be Areas' future manpower requirements.

In order to formulate a view on the likely future manpower situation
for monitoring purposes manpower planners at Regional level had to
undertake two major analyses. The first attempted to quantify the
numbers and types of staff the Region and Areas would require in 1981
and 1988, in order to estimate Areas' possible targets in the different
professions and skills of manpower. The second tried to quantify how
much of this target could be achieved through the available resource
assumptions in order to note likely shortfalls in staff and the effects
of changes in priorities between the expansion of one staff group and
another.

By concentrating on an assessment of future additional requirements
for staff in the different professions and skills, and contrasting it
with a projection of present spending policies on the staff groups, the
analysis helped to identify the need for new manpower policies during
the plan period or changes in existing ones. Such assessments would
allow greater direction, accuracy and confidence in allocating revenue
and in planning the training and recruitment of staff, as well as
identifying any continuing deprivation in staffing due to the lack of
revenue resources or staff availability. The objective was to give an
indication of what the Region felt they would have attained in terms of
staffing in 1981 and 1988. In the absence of a true definition of
requirements through service development and due to time constraints it
was decided to adopt the methodology of projecting national average
rates of staffing to 1988 and then attempt to compare them with the
likely constraints of revenue resources.

The projected national average staffing levels were based upon
projections in relation to population; in the case of Areas the same
populations were used to formulate the revenue assumptions. In the
past, and indeed for the last round of strategic plans, these national
average staffing projections had been made on the basis of historical
trends in staffing in the absence of any better method. For this
analysis growth rates were based on an initial investigation by the DHSS
Manpower Intelligence Branch of the desired movement in programme
budgets nationally and thus changes in staffing resulting from it. The
analysis went as far as was presently possible from a Regional level in
seeking to describe the requirements for additional manpower during the
plan period. It was not designed to be, and could not replace, a true
identification of demand for manpower through service development.

Projected national averages had been attempted in one form or another
before. Even if the requirements for additional manpower could be
perfectly defined they would still not be realistic unless related to
the amount of revenue available to employ additional staff. In order
to give the Region some indication of the extent to which the demand for
manpower was likely to be achieved it was decided to attempt to relate
the projected national average levels to available finance. Regional
officers did not feel that they were in a position to describe the

manner in which each Area would seek to spend its additional revenue resources as this was very much an issue for local policy making. The objective of the analysis was to identify those professions and skills where the projected requirements for manpower would not be met due to lack of finance. It was therefore decided to allocate additional Area revenue to the staffing groups in the same way as actually happened in the financial year 1976/77. By the use of such a financial breakdown, admittedly in rough and ready terms, the effect of the projected additional revenue resources on levels of staffing was identified. It was decided that these analyses could also be useful to Areas as parameters against which they could test their plans. Further refinements in the analyses were later carried out to update the projected national averages with new data on the likely growth rates in staffing from the DHSS Manpower Intelligence Branch and to note how staffing numbers would differ if national expenditure patterns rather than Regional ones were used to constrain manpower growth within the finance available.

Discussion

The eventual production of Area strategic plans was both an encouragement and a disappointment to Regional manpower planners. On the one hand, manpower played a much greater role in all plans than it did in 1976. On the other hand, no one Area was able to provide a comprehensive manpower strategy as required by the planning system. It was found that in most plans the Region could attempt to assess the conformity of staffing proposals within financial projections, even though some Area strategies proved to be well wide of their financial constraints. An assessment of medical and nursing staff proposals by service group was also possible. It was obvious that Areas were not setting priorities for development within the manpower strategy and most plans were akin to a shopping list. A true identification of future demand had not been carried out based on the Area strategy for service development. Despite the emphasis given to standardisation and the completion of SASP forms in the Regional guidance this had not been adhered to and different gaps in the manpower strategy were found in the different Area plans.

The formulation of the manpower element of the Regional strategic plan has had to be more than a mere compilation of Area plans. The future demand for staff has been entirely based on Area plans. In cases where an Area has not provided a demand figure the manpower planners have used the monitoring analyses to do so. The manpower demand strategy basically conforms with the likely financial limitations. But in very few cases did Area plans make an attempt to gauge the likely supply of staff available to them or the consequences of a lack of supply, or formulate policies intended to curb this constraint on service development. It can be argued that the Region is better placed to formulate policy on the supply of staff, especially those who are professionally trained by the service for the service. In any case, Regional manpower planners felt that the manpower strategy would not be complete without attempting an assessment of likely supply trends and policies to affect them.

By analysing past wastage patterns it was possible to assess the total numbers of staff who would need to be recruited in the future to replace

120

leavers and accomplish the development required by the manpower strategy. Against this figure for each profession, sub-profession and staff group could be put the past recruitment record. The analysis was therefore able to state that, although 'X' was the level of recruitment in the past, 'Y' needed to be the level of recruitment in the future. Such an analysis gave basic pointers to where the supply of staff was likely to fall short of requirements or, in certain staff groups, considerably exceed them. The Regional manpower strategy was therefore able to note potential problems of supply, give priority to future detailed analysis, and point towards actions to remedy these situations.

It is difficult to assess what effect the attempt to assist Areas had upon their plans. Better manpower strategies were produced than had been the case in 1976. This may have been a natural progression and something which would have happened without the Region's assistance. But it is unlikely that plans would have conformed to a set pattern without the work carried out in the monitoring analyses. There would not have been as much quantification of manpower demand, nor would the Region have been in a position to fill in the gaps in Areas' manpower strategies. However, perhaps a direct result of such involvement has been the greater communication which has resulted between Area and Region on manpower planning matters. This has included the inception of a quarterly meeting of Area and Regional manpower planners to encourage the interchange and development of information, to act as a focus for training and education, to ensure a better administration of and focus for manpower planning activity, and to operate as a forum for generating ideas on the future development of manpower planning in the Region. In some ways the group is modelled on MAPLIN (6) and fulfils the same functions on a Regional scale.

Conclusion

It is too early to pass judgement on the recent planning round. However, some lessons have been learnt in Trent which will undoubtedly affect the future development of manpower planning in the Region and, as part of that, the next round of strategic planning scheduled for 1982. There has been a questionmark over the appropriate location of manpower planning activity. The basic belief in planning in Trent is that strategies on the development of the service can only be adequately produced at local level. There is no alternative in the 'real world' to bottom up planning, but to achieve it requires a long term process of development of a planning consciousness in the mind of every manager in the service. Managers must gain the ability not only to assess the needs of today but to look forward and plan for them before they materialise. In terms of manpower this means that the future demand for staff can only be assessed at or near District level. An overall analysis is not feasible due to widely differing claims placed on the service, the different skill mixes of staff that result, and the different conditions within which staff function. There is, however, little capacity at the operational level to affect the supply of manpower. Much of the co-ordination of supply, the institutions of training and development lie at Regional and national levels. Communication between levels must be improved in order to co-ordinate these two basic elements of the manpower equation in a timely and effective manner.

The willingness of local management to recognise and develop their role in manpower planning is crucial. Part of the reason for a specialist manpower planning role at Regional level was the necessity to educate, advise and assist local management and act as a source of data and technical expertise. The inception of the meetings of Area and Regional manpower planners plays a major part in developing this role. Planning and manpower planning cannot and should not be seen as exercises which happen once in four years for the strategic plan, and annually for the operational plan. Planning is a continual process, the plan just being a periodic culmination of planning activity. It is planning that must be promoted, not the written plan.

There has been much criticism of national (and Regional) guidance on which plans are meant to be based. This is not a criticism of the political, Civil Service, or NHS administrative machinery. It is rather the realisation that, as planning can only be accomplished bottom up by assessing and voicing the needs of the service from the patient upwards, and as this has not yet been accomplished by the planning system, there is little for national policy makers to work on to provide guidance on priorities. It is perhaps not surprising that the service is so short of realistic manpower policies.

A CASE STUDY OF WESSEX RHA

P. Dixon and J. Cree

Introduction

The recent introduction of strategic planning and the requirement for a corporate approach to this process has presented a difficult challenge to all those concerned with the planning of manpower. Considering that of the total revenue expenditure of the NHS more than 70 per cent is spent on staff - this amounted to approximately £170 million in Wessex during the 1978/79 financial year - the attention paid to the planning of the service's largest resource has been scant. The NHS is still struggling to identify valid relationships between the health services provided and the staff required to operate these services and to increase the understanding of the behaviour and characteristics of its manpower through the improvement and development of relevant information systems.

Because of the size of the manpower resource in the NHS together with the variety of professions and occupations, each with their own training and career requirements, manpower planning effort has tended to be concentrated on fairly detailed studies of individual staff groups. (7) The increasing financial restrictions imposed on the NHS, together with a growing realisation that there is not going to be an endless supply of suitable manpower, are now focusing attention on the need to look carefully at the total picture: to estimate the full implications for all staff groups of the service being planned for the future and to search for alternative means of providing these services if either money or manpower supply are seen to be inadequate. The importance of treating manpower as one of the primary resources of the NHS, central to the continued existence of a comprehensive health service, is at last being realised.

At a time of limited resources and of increasing pressures to improve the efficiency of the services provided, as well as trying to implement national policies for the development of the 'Cinderella' services, (8) strategic planning assumes a critical role. No longer can NHS managers continue to apply the incremental approach to the development of services. They are forced to examine alternatives as to how increasing and changing demands for care can be met with the same, if not less, resources available. Central to this process are the questions surrounding manpower: what sort and how many staff are needed; can they be funded; could they be recruited; what training is needed; and so on. If feasible solutions to any identified manpower problems cannot be found then alternative ways of staffing planned services have to be examined. If all else fails, the service plans themselves may have to be amended. Even from this brief description of the questions to be asked about manpower one can see the size of the exercise. Nor is it a one-off process; every plan must be tested and amended regularly as knowledge and environments change. (9)

The approach described here to long term manpower planning has concentrated on ensuring a means by which the vital manpower questions can be asked and the possible solutions integrated into a total, corporate plan for the future investment of capital, revenue and

manpower. Central to the approach to strategic planning taken in
Wessex are two beliefs: the objectives for care must be translated into
their resource implications; and each of the resources available to the
NHS has implications for all the others. For example, capital
investment cannot be planned in isolation from manpower and revenue, nor
can the implications of a change in basic training requirements be
identified without reference to the effects on service provision,
financial allocations or physical accommodation.

Background to planning in Wessex

Before describing how Wessex attempted to integrate manpower with the
planning of all other resources it is useful to outline the history
behind the strategic plan in Wessex and to describe the overall
structure of the plan. The Wessex Region has had a planning system in
operation since 1974 and, despite innumerable teething problems,
planning is becoming an integral part of management. Planning was,
however, mainly limited to capital developments with only tentative
attempts to plan for the provision of services in total. The manpower
contributions to these plans were scarce, held only tenuous links with
the capital plans, and did not take financial constraints into account.
Over the last two years the emphasis has changed. The importance of a
corporate planning process has been recognised together with the need
for a team approach to planning at Regional level. Service, capital,
manpower, and financial planners who had previously operated in
isolation were forced together to develop an integrated framework which
incorporated all the various aspects of the health service.

  The work required to achieve this integration has been considerable
and some long cherished ideas for the development of techniques within
each of these specialist disciplines have had to be sacrificed for the
good of the whole. In terms of manpower planning two major problems
had to be overcome. Firstly, as the service plans were to be expressed
in terms of care groups, (10) the integration of manpower and service
plans necessitated a care group analysis of manpower. As there was no
available means of classifying staff in this way an apportionment
procedure was adopted through the development of a computer model.
Secondly, there had to be a means of linking the manpower predictions to
revenue. It was felt that as the manpower forecasts were based upon
service proposals, and as manpower expenditure was known to consume a
large proportion of the available revenue each year, then a future
revenue investment programme for each care group could be derived from
the manpower projections. The means by which this was achieved is
described in the section on manpower methodology.

  The actual structure of the plan also had considerable implications
for the ways in which the manpower input had to be made. The approach
taken in Wessex was that a plan ought to start with a statement of the
objective of the organisation. A plan is a considered statement of the
intended actions and these actions must have a direction - a goal.
Unless the Region can identify where it wishes to go it is impossible to
plan how to get there. The goal was defined as the sum of the Regional
aims and policies for particular services together with the standards of
provision to achieve these aims. The level of facilities required to
achieve the goal was called the service goal and did not take into
account existing buildings or patterns of service in the Region. In

other words, the setting of the service goal was based upon the concept that if the Region was just embarking upon the task of building up a health service from scratch, then how would a comprehensive health service, provided to a good standard in every District, be defined? The resources needed to achieve the service goal were then measured in terms of capital, revenue and manpower.

The next stage was the analysis of current levels of provision. A comparison of the existing situation with the goal gave an indication of the shortfall. The identification of the shortfall in this way provided the Region with measures of relative deficiency which were central to the subsequent analysis of priorities for future investment. For example, the absolute shortfall for the acute services is three times that for services for the elderly. One approach to the planning of future investment would therefore argue that the priority for the development of services should be in the acute sector. Looking at the relative deficiencies, however, the acute shortfall represents 33 per cent of the existing level of provision whilst the shortfall in the elderly sector represents a 50 per cent deficiency. The examination of relative deficiencies was selected by Wessex as the most appropriate means by which judgements on priorities could be made. Along side the examination of priorities a number of constraints which would affect progress towards the goal were identified. One obvious constraint was finance; but others, such as the availability of manpower and the social, economic and political climate had also to be taken into consideration.

Taking into account the interaction of the goals, shortfalls, priorities and constraints previously identified, the Region went on to examine options for investment which were within the resources predicted and which would ensure progress towards the goal. The option seen to be the one which would being the service closest to its goals in the period was selected and expressed as a series of investment targets (in terms of capital, revenue and manpower) and policy statements. The strategy to be followed to enable the targets to be met in practical terms was then set out.

Manpower methodology

Each stage of the plan had to be expressed in terms of the service provision translated into the resources required - capital, revenue and manpower. In addition, the services and resources were to be classified by care group or programme as set out in Figure 20 of the DHSS planning guide. In terms of the manpower element a complicated matrix of numerous staff occupations and nine different care groups was confronted, all to be examined within the context of each AHA within the Region.

The first step was to decide upon a classification of manpower which was manageable and yet sufficiently detailed to be meaningful for planning purposes. With this in mind, the first time that the planning methods were put into practice and tested (in 1977) the total regional workforce was divided only into the six main Whitley divisions of staff; namely, medical and dental, nursing, administrative and clerical, building and engineering, professional and technical, and ancillary. In 1978, as methods were refined and confidence increased,

the manpower classification was expanded to 16 staffing groups.   For
example, the original nursing category was subdivided into qualified,
unqualified and learner nurses.

The classifications agreed, the process of working through the various
stages of the plan was initiated.   The first stage in the strategic
plan was to define the Regional goal and to translate the improvements
for the provision of health services into the facilities required (beds,
day places, health centres, and so on) to derive the service goal.
Whilst the service goal took no account of current levels of service,
the measurement of the resources required to achieve it drew upon
experiences gained from existing practices and levels of provision.
If established norms or yardsticks had been available, either within the
Region or nationally (for example, a recommended number of nurses per
acute bed), such ratios would have been used.   In the absence of such
yardsticks Regional staffing standards had to be developed from an
examination of current staff to service ratios.

The manpower forecasts were therefore based upon an analysis of
existing stock.   The first step in this process was to achieve a care
group classification of manpower, a classification demanded by the
planning system but not readily achievable in manpower terms.   None of
the existing methods of classifying staff lends itself to a care group
analysis. (11)   Discounting the possibilities of a lengthy and
expensive questionnaire or local form filling exercise (which could
never be expected to be repeated on a regular basis for monitoring
purposes), it was decided to develop an apportionment method based upon
information readily available at Region.

The method developed was based upon an analysis of the services
provided, the manpower employed and the expenditure on both staff and
non staffing items at hospital level.   The process hinged upon the
ability to classify accurately the services and facilities at each
hospital by care group and then to make assumptions about the relationship of manpower and expenditure to those services in order to derive an
estimate of the investment made in each care group of staff and revenue.
The final result of this existing analysis was to achieve an estimate of
the number and cost of each staff category by care group within each
Authority and for the Region as a whole, and to derive a similar
analysis of total revenue expenditure.   It was never intended as a
totally accurate representation of manpower and revenue investment but
rather as a broad brush tool which provided a sufficiently valid
baseline for strategic planning.

The advantage for manpower planning in this approach was that the
combination of service, financial and staffing data allowed for the
calculation of a variety of manpower ratios which, in the absence of
acceptable national or local manpower standards, could be used as a
basis for forecasts.   Examples of the relationships resulting from this
analysis of the existing state were the number of staff per facility
provided in a care group (nurses per bed); the number of staff per head
of population (community midwives per 1,000 female population); the
average cost of employing a number of staff of a particular staff group
within a care group; and the proportion of total revenue spent on staff
within each care group.   Such ratios or standards were then used as a
basis for examining the requirements for change as expressed in the

manpower goal.

The setting of the manpower goal had to be done within the corporate objectives of the Region and means had to be found for translating these objectives into manpower requirements. At the same time, other factors which were likely to uniquely affect the manpower resource had to be identified and built into the forecasts. The Regional objectives were firstly expressed in terms of services, and the physical facilities required to provide such services to a goal standard. These facilities, in terms of their type, quantity and location, obviously had implications for manpower but the manpower forecasts could not simply be the result of applying existing staffing standards to a revised estimate of future capital stock (service goal). There was an obvious need to assess the existing levels of manpower provision and, where necessary, to define required changes. In addition there are categories of service not linked to capital stock and there are certain staff groups, such as medical and dental, who are required to provide a service to the population as a whole, not just to those attending a health institution.

The manpower forecasts for the goal were, therefore, based upon an examination of the existing staffing standards, the assessment of those factors which should or would have an impact on those standards in the future, and the quantification of the effect of such factors. The implications of changes in hospital throughput, changes in population size and structure, technological advances, changes to working hours and changes in emphasis of care were all examined and discussed with the professions. In particular, efforts were made to comply with national and Regional objectives for improvement in standards of care in the long stay and community fields.

The results of this analysis were quantified in terms of percentage increases to the existing staffing standards to produce goal staffing standards. For example, the existing ratio in the acute care group may have been one nurse per bed. The combined effects of forecasts of a shorter working week, an increase in throughput per bed and an increase in patient dependency could be estimated to cause a requirement for an increase of 30 per cent on the existing ratio to give a goal nursing standard of 1.3 nurses per acute bed. The goal standards were applied to the service goal to obtain estimates of the total numbers of staff required to run the services in 1988 at these levels. The staff numbers were then costed by the application of the average costs derived from the existing analysis. Finally, through assumptions made on how the staff/non staff expenditure relationship might change, the total revenue required to run the services at goal levels was derived (the revenue goal in Figure 7.1, p.129).

The costs, both capital and revenue, required to meet the service goal were expected to be in excess of the finances forecast to be available, and a means of deciding on optimum investment patterns, taking into account the various priorities and constraints, had to be found. For this purpose a 'targetting process' was developed which was based on the principle that each Area Authority and each care group within it should reach the same position relative to its service goal at the end of the plan period. Various options for investment were explored to assess the effect on the pattern of resource allocation of changing assumptions about priorities, resources available, transfer of funds between capital and revenue, and so on, and one option selected as the 'best fit'. The manpower implications of the preferred option were derived by constraining the goal staffing levels in each Authority and each care group within the revenue available.

This description of the manpower methodology has of necessity been fairly superficial. Each stage of the method - the analysis of the existing state, the setting of goal staffing standards, the manpower results of the targetting process - could be discussed at great length. In this paper an attempt has been made to describe the principles of the approach adopted. Figure 7.1 summarises the methods used for deriving the manpower forecasts, and highlights the main stages: analysing the existing state of services, manpower and revenue expenditure; combining the results of this analysis to produce goal staffing standards; applying these goal standards to the service goal; costing the manpower results; and finally constraining the goals within the limits of the finance likely to be available to the Region.

Discussion

Much effort has been concentrated in this approach on the development of a methodology which will allow a variety of views of the future to be tested out and the implications of these views quantified in terms of all resources. The capital and service elements are well advanced but the manpower contribution is still at an embryonic stage. However, several important steps forward have been achieved.

Firstly, the methodology has firmly established manpower as an integral and essential part of the strategic plan. The links between the service plans and the resources required to achieve those plans together with the inter-relationship between the resource of capital money, revenue and manpower show the beginnings of a corporate approach to planning. Any change to the service requirement can be readily converted into the implications of this change on the required resources. Any change to the supply or demand for any one resource can be followed through to calculate the effects this would have on other resources.

Secondly, the plan has legitimised the use of value judgements and has allowed the implications of these value judgements to be quantified and tested. Developments in the health service have taken place in the past without the explicit direction and control of a strategic plan. This process of development has been based largely upon the intuition and experience of individual managers. The methodology developed in Wessex has forced these intuitions, or value judgements, to be made explicit. Assumptions can then be challenged and adopted openly which must aid the development of an improved health service.

Thirdly, perhaps the most important result has been that the manpower plan has initiated interest and debate on manpower issues and has paved the way for the future development of manpower planning. The method has provided a framework on to which the results of further, more detailed, manpower investigations can be latched and the implications followed through in terms of their impact on other planned developments.

One fundamental danger inherent in the method adopted which has

Fig 7.1 *A summary of the Manpower Methodology*

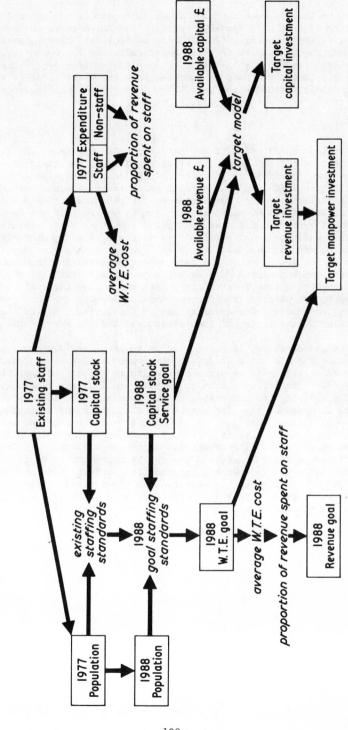

already become apparent within the Wessex Region is the natural desire amongst managers for a tangible set of criteria on which to base their actions. The existence of a national or Regional staffing standard, or norm, may cause managers to avoid questioning the appropriateness of using that standard within their own specific environment. The philosophy behind the manpower component of the Wessex plan is that it only provides a foundantion upon which individual authorities can build up their own manpower scenarios.

Conclusion

The manpower contribution to the strategic plan was basically an estimate of the total number of staff required in the tenth year to run the services specified in the plan at a Regional normative level. It was not a specification of the total recruitment necessary as no account was taken of turnover. For instance, the plan identified a need for a net increase of 10,000 staff in the next 10 years. If the Region had an average turnover of 10 per cent per annum, then over 10 years 50,000 new staff would be required simply to maintain existing staff levels. Thus in future years a detailed examination of internal supply is essential before comprehensive recruitment and training programmes can be formulated and costed. A second major area for development must be an investigation into whether the Region can manage the scale of change implied by the plan. The manpower implications of the proposed closures, openings and changes in use of facilities could be a serious constraint on the timing or even achievement of the service plans.

The method developed is now available to Areas and Districts within the Region who wish to identify the manpower implications of service plans and to test out assumptions relating to changes in manpower standards. The enormous data collection and analysis problems have been lifted from them and they can now concentrate on the important aspects of manpower planning; that is, the setting of objectives, the testing of assumptions, and the planning of actions required to achieve their objectives. This is already proving to be the most difficult problem that the Wessex approach has encountered. The need for authorities to fully understand the implications of the Regional plan and to utilise the framework it provides to produce their own plans is a far greater challenge than was originally perceived. There is clearly going to be a learning period for both the Region and the Districts before the full potential of the planning methods are realised.

NOTES

(1)   The data discussed here relate to replies to a postal questionnaire administered in June 1979 to Regional focal points in manpower planning in England.   Completed returns were obtained from 12 of the 14 persons. The survey data have been reported elsewhere.   See, A.F.Long and G.Mercer, 'Manpower Planning in the NHS - A Report of a Survey', Nuffield Centre for Health Services Studies, University of Leeds, April 1980;   and A.F.Long and G.Mercer, 'NHS Manpower Planning - Towards a Positive Approach?', Health Services Manpower Review, vol.6, nos.2 and 3, 1980.
(2)   For example, Resource Allocation Working Party (RAWP), Sharing Resources for Health in England, HMSO, London 1976.
(3)   DHSS, The Way Forward, HMSO, London 1977.
(4)   Trent Regional Health Authority, 'Regional Guidelines for Strategic Planning 1978/9', Trent Regional Health Authority, April 1978.
(5)   See, DHSS, The NHS Planning System, HC(76)30, DHSS, London 1976, Figure 20, and as revised in, 'Strategic Planning in 1978: Planning Manual', DHSS letter from R.S.King to Regional administrators, January 1978.
(6)   For details on MAPLIN, see R.Petch, 'The Role of the DHSS', Chapter Six of this volume.
(7)   For example, see the following reports: Department of Education and Science, Speech Therapy Services, (Quirk Report), HMSO, London 1972; DHSS, Recruitment and Training of Dental Hygienists, (Interim Report), HMSO, London 1974; Health Services Organisation Research Unit, Brunel University, 'Organisation of Physiotherapy and Occupational Therapy in the NHS', Working Paper, 1977.
(8)   DHSS, Priorities for Health and Personal Social Services in England, A Consultative Document, HMSO, London 1976.
(9)   DHSS, The NHS Planning System.
(10) Ibid., Figure 20, Annex 1.
(11) Existing manpower information systems allow for the classification of staff by grade, professional group, occupation, location and function (pathology, laundry and so on).   There is no coding structure currently available by which all staff can be classified by care group. For a discussion of manpower information systems, see J.Cree, 'A Manpower Information System', Chapter Four of this volume.

8 Devolution: The Role of the Local Level

A. F. Long and G. Mercer

Manpower planning in the NHS has been typically carried out at a
national level by the DHSS through committees of enquiry and
commissions. (1)   It has tended to focus on one side of the manpower
equation, specifically to assist decision making on the size of student
intakes.   A key role has been played in medical manpower planning,
especially on the supply side, and in disseminating norms and guidelines
to the NHS. (2)   More recently, Regional Health Authorities have
nominated an officer as the Regional focal point on manpower planning,
following DHSS' decision to broaden the membership of MAPLIN and to
encourage actively the development of manpower planning within the NHS.
(3)   Some RHAs have developed specific manpower planning units (within
personnel) whilst in others it is almost a one person unit within or
outside the personnel division.   The Region's emerging role has
revolved around giving advice and assistance to the local health
authorities in formulating the manpower component of strategic plans.
(4)   So far, few Area Health Authorities have assigned an officer
solely to manpower planning, leaving it to the personnel and planning
functions to sort out.   Indeed, the role of the Area and District is
clouded with uncertainty.

   This chapter attempts to explore the tasks and responsibilities of the
local health authority in manpower planning.   The first section
examines the arguments of two recent commentators on manpower planning
in the NHS: Stocking, who puts forward the case for a more centralised
manpower planning function;   and the Merrison Report, which supports its
devolution, except for the medical and dental practitioners. (5)   The
underlying issue is whether manpower planning should be centralised or
devolved to the lowest level in the NHS structure where it can still be
tackled effectively.   Earlier contributors to this volume have
indicated the directional role of the centre and the Regional tier.
The tasks and responsibilities of the local level remain to be
amplified.   In consequence, the second section looks at current
practice of manpower planning at the Area and District level through an
examination of fieldwork undertaken by the authors in 1979.   It
explores the awareness of manpower as a resource within planning and the
way the manpower input to planning was drawn up.   The chapter concludes
with a discussion of the role of the various tiers from DHSS to the
District in manpower planning.

Stocking raises the issue of whether manpower planning could take place at a local or Regional level for staff 'complementary' to medicine. (6) According to her perspective, the argument is not so much about devolution as logistics.   On the supply side, for several of the non medical professions, the numbers required are so small as to make local manpower planning impossible.   There is also the problem of over production in one Region and its effect on other parts of the NHS.   On the demand side, total funds for the NHS and priorities are decided nationally.   In addition, the demand for trained staff manpower is the sum total of decisions by employing authorities.   Accordingly, she argues, there is a need for 'some central body piecing together the total picture to assess what the overall requirement is and will be.' (7)   Devolution is thus not the aim, but rather further centralisation, even for the larger professions such as nursing. (8)   In other words, all manpower planning for trained staff, doctors and their complementary professions has to be carried out centrally.

In contrast, the report of the Royal Commission on the NHS came out in July 1979 with the following conclusion: '. . . the needs and resources of different parts of the UK varied so greatly that centralised planning for all NHS staff would be wholly impracticable . . . An exception to this is medical and dental manpower . . .' (9)   To understand this argument, it is necessary to look back at the committee's perceptions of the key problems on the manpower planning front.   Two broad aspects were perceived: firstly, estimating total numbers needed; and secondly, getting such staff to the right places.   Many central efforts have been directed to getting an appropriate distribution of doctors in the NHS, while training and recruitment have been carried out locally, for the majority of NHS staff.   The latter arrangement '. . . leaves the management function of manpower planning largely to health authorities and the function of estimating numbers largely in abeyance. It has the advantage of flexibility.' (10)   This flexibility is interpreted by others as a recipe for inaction, more especially because it does not clarify who is to do what.   In contrast, medical manpower planning needs an elaborate central machinery '. . . to direct (doctors) to specialities and areas where they are needed.' (11)

The Merrison committee addressed itself directly to the proposal for a central planning body '. . . with the function of assessing the numbers and types of staff required for the NHS and the implications for the educational system.' (12)   In the members' view, such a body would have little to contribute to what they saw as the main difficulty in the NHS, '. . . ensuring the proper distribution of its workers.   In our view this must remain the business of health departments and the health authorities.' (13)   It would also be a force for centralisation where in fact it is necessary for authorities '. . . to recruit and train the staff they need within an overall policy.' (14)   They conclude that '. . . while we do not advocate new central manpower planning bodies, we do consider that a more positive approach to manpower planning generally is required.' (15)

Neither of these perspectives makes explicit the role that each health authority should play nor exactly how the centre should carry out its preeminent responsibility.   Stocking is no doubt correct in arguing

that there is a role for a central body to put together the total
picture on manpower. It is perhaps in this light that the 'SASP' table
on manpower, to be completed as part of the strategic plan and focusing
on current and future staffing levels four and 10 years on, can be seen
as communicating the raw data. (16) The problem lies in what a central
body should do beyond this. Here the Merrison Report gives an
indication, but only for medical and dental staff - to assess demand and
fix training and education levels. This covers only a part of the area
of manpower planning. It leaves aside the question of alternative
sources of supply, apart from teaching school outputs (for example, the
'pool' of potential qualified recruits); begs the question of how much
influence a central body could have on the local supply (and thus
distribution) of manpower; and fails to answer the question of how
demand for manpower can be assessed at a central level.

Both commentators agree that medical manpower planning needs to be
undertaken at the centre. Merrison highlights the long training time,
high expense, and the involvement of the universities as the basic
reasons. (17) As the Regional administrators suggested in evidence to
the Royal Commission, 'the key to the redeployment of manpower resources
in the NHS is the redeployment of medical staff, for the necessary
support in terms of other professional staff will follow providing the
financial resources are likewise redeployed.' (18) Efforts in the past
to redistribute medical resources seem hardly to have had much effect
despite DHSS efforts. Perhaps the new procedures on resource
allocation outlined in the RAWP report will have greater impact. (19)
Indeed such are the experiences and hopes expressed in 'RAWP gaining'
Regions such as Trent. (20) However, on past evidence, central
manpower planning fixes training numbers and only marginally influences
the redistribution of manpower. It must be remembered, though, that
other levels in the NHS can influence, at least potentially, the supply
of medical staff. Strategies such as intra-professional contact, the
rearrangement of working hours to suit returning (part time) female
staff, and even the substitution of staff or the direction of newly
trained staff to areas of need could be employed by the local health
authorities themselves to effect in order to overcome supply
difficulties. (21)

In addition, Stocking argued that a centralised manpower planning body
is required to consider professions 'complementary to medicine'.
Several comments must be made. Firstly, while it is true that for
paramedical groups such as speech therapists or chiropodists the numbers
involved are small even at a Regional level, this is not the case for
groups such as occupational therapists, radiographers, and the biggest
health profession of all, nurses. Indeed, it could be argued that
'local' manpower planning is essential to ensure that sufficient numbers
are trained at least to meet local needs. Secondly, for medical,
nursing and paramedical groups, the broader question of the training
school 'constituency' has to be thought through and resolved: is it for
the profession, the funding body, or the Region, Area or District where
the school is located? Finally, Stocking appears to exaggerate the
pivotal role of the DHSS in controlling the NHS. In contrast, the NHS
spends its monies in the context of centrally generated and locally
interpreted priorities. The planning system is itself explicitly
bottom up. (22) The argument against the devolution of manpower
planning is thus questionable for many staff groups, especially where

the labour market is Regional, and more so where it is local.   It also
ignores the potential and actual influences over the demand and supply
of manpower open to local health authorities, as well as the fact that
the manpower issues faced at the various levels in the NHS differ
within and across staff group.   For example, it is at a local
divisional level that nurse sickness and absence is a critical issue, as
are questions of selecting the right person for the job.   This is also
the case for paramedical staff.   The numbers of nurses to train must be
raised at the (Area) Authority level, while for paramedics and doctors
training requirements have to be resolved higher up the organisation.

   In arguing in favour of the devolution of manpower planning, the
Merrison Report mentions that the central health departments have a role
to play in monitoring '. . . the quality of the treatment and care
provided by NHS workers, and (if possible) . . . to lay down staff
norms, to forecast needs and deficiencies, and eliminate shortages.'
(23)   It did not, however, explore the implications of devolution for
manpower planning practice and responsibilities.   Its sole emphasis lay
on the area of recruitment.   'Recruitment decisions should, for the
most part, be made locally in the light of local needs within an overall
policy.' (24)   Many gaps and question marks remain: who is to explore
the supply side and training, and within whose overall policy?   Further
weight behind the trend towards devolution was provided by the
reorganisation of the NHS in 1974 and by the consultative document
Patients First in 1979. (25)   'We are determined to see that as many
decisions as possible are taken at the local level . . . We are
determined to have more local health authorities, whose members will be
encouraged to manage the Service with the minimum of interference by any
central authority, whether at region or in central government departments.' (26)

   In the argument that the devolution of manpower planning in the NHS is
desirable, the local health authority emerges with a heightened
contribution.   The contention is not that there is no role for a
central tier, but that lower levels in the organisation (the Area and
District, or new District Health Authority) can and must perform part of
the task.   Indeed, the strategic centre, irrespective of whether it is
the Region or the DHSS, would be primarily involved in co-ordinating and
monitoring, rather than detailed planning or implementation.   What then
is the role to be played by the local level?   Part of the answer can be
gleaned from looking at the planning system and from exploring the
manpower planning equation itself, specifically where the demand for
manpower is generated and its supply located.   The further issue of
potential influences authorities could exert over the demand and supply
of staff is explored in Chapter Nine.

   To carry out the roles required in the planning system, it is
obligatory that authorities give consideration to manpower. (27)
Indeed, for (Regional and Area) strategic planning the SASP manpower
table has to be completed.   For operational planning, the manpower
element, focusing on such things as the redeployment of staff from one
location to another, achievement of staff recruitment and the longer
term implications for staff training, (28) is of fundamental importance.
It is within operational planning itself that the likelihood of
achieving requisite manpower supply, and thus of meeting the strategic
plan within the indicated timescale, will be examined.   District

operational plans are pieces in the Region's jigsaw, indicating in the short term how the longer term Regional strategy is to be implemented. Within strategic planning supply constraints may only affect the time scale over which the plan will be implemented and not the overall direction services should move in.

Of greater importance for manpower planning itself is the issue of 'integration'. Manpower planning in the NHS has been characterised by its concentration on one staff group at a time. For example, the recent DHSS consultative document on medical manpower planning does not consider the question of the implications of altering the number of doctors on other health staff groups. (29) From reflecting upon the essential function that nurses, remedial and scientific professions play in the provision of health services, the limitations of a uni-disciplinary perspective can be seen. It is important to develop manpower planning not by discipline, but rather across discipline and staff groups, identifying the most appropriate mixes of staff to provide patient care. The objective of health manpower planning must be '. . . to specify the number of (health) teams and the composition needed to improve the level of health . . .' (30) The planning link is through the development of a care group approach to health services planning, where the activities are centred upon examining and designing services for 'client' or care groups, such as the elderly or children. (31)

Co-ordinated manpower planning across disciplines is an innovation that the planning system could foster. Changing demand for nurses, for example, is not simply a direct response to medical expansion or contraction. They are related to each other and to developments in other staff groups; but, most importantly, they are both based on patient/service needs. At issue is the mix of staff required to provide the appropriate services for the care group, rather than the straightforward application of manpower to population ratios as bases for estimates of the demand. (32) It is primarily at the local level that such an integrated approach can be generated. The link into the planning system is immediate - the consideration of service targets, ways to achieve them, and the manpower consequences. Determination of supply is relevant in raising the issues of the necessary substitution of less trained for trained staff, or role enlargement to cover shortages in a skilled area. Higher levels in the organisation may then only need to consider and summarise total staff requirements by staff group, leaving to the local level questions over manpower demand in relation to patient/service needs, and the ultimate manpower distribution.

The demand for manpower, irrespective of staff group skill, mix or grades, tends to be generated at the local level. Within the NHS planning system demands arise either from an examination of current service provision and service objectives and/or from the implementation of guidance from a higher tier - Area, Region and even the DHSS. Whatever the source there is a critical role to be played by the departmental manager, be it the head of occupational therapy, the divisional nurse, or the consultant. While in an ideal world estimates of manpower requirements should arise from an examination of the population's needs (as defined by the patient and clinician), in practice resort is made to the application of manpower to population ratios and, particularly where these are lacking, to subjective estimates of demands on the department and manpower appropriate to provide the service at a given level and standard.

Turning to the supply side of manpower, the situation is equally complex. Again, no one level has sole influence or control. The labour market for manpower varies in relation to the staff group in question, and the grades of staff within it. For example, among nursing assistants the local environment to the hospital concerned is the likely labour market, whereas for staff nurses and ward sisters it broadens to at least the District (if it is geographically self-contained) or to other Districts within the same AHA or to another AHA. Furthermore, different labour markets apply to potential recruits for training (nursing, medicine, radiography, and so on) and for actual job vacancies. Finally, there is variation in the stability (and thus the flows both out of the NHS and within it) of staff groups and grades, affecting the frequency with which one has to return to the labour market for 'additional supply'. In other words, the supply of manpower is not centred within one location or one labour market. Concern over the supply of manpower and ways of influencing it are, therefore, likely to range from the District level right across and up to the Region, and even to the inter-Regional level.

It is no simple solution to devolve manpower planning respons-ibilities. On the one hand, each level in the NHS from the DHSS to the District has a role to play and influences to wield over the demand and supply of manpower. For example, to argue that the shorter the duration of training the greater the influence or control the District has over supply is to minimise many potential avenues of influence. Nevertheless, some options are more open and more effective than others due to such factors as professional interest and control, and trade union concern. On the other hand, the integrated, care group approach to manpower planning and the planning roles of the various levels both emphasise the role of the local health authorities in manpower planning. From the planning system itself, the pull is towards the need for a heightened role for the local health authority, while remembering that each level has its part to play; the tiers are not independent, but interdependent.

MANPOWER PLANNING PRACTICE AT THE LOCAL LEVEL

The previous discussion has explored the issue of the centralisation or devolution of manpower planning and highlighted the important role of the local health authorities in manpower planning. Its part in formulating demand for manpower and affecting supply and in pioneering an integrated (care group) approach to manpower planning have been stressed. Attention now turns to examine how Area and District health authorities are actually carrying out manpower planning. A sample survey investigation undertaken by the authors in 1979 provides the basis for the discussion. (33) Interviews were conducted and postal questionnaires administered to personnel and planning officers in selected areas and districts in five regions in England. In all, the survey respondents relate to 12 AHAs (including three single district areas) and 12 districts. The concern was to obtain responses on a broad and representative basis.

It should be pointed out that while 44 local health authorities were approached only 24 replied. From comments received by the researchers it became clear that some of the respondents perceived the focus of the questionnaire as a threat, exploring an area where a key role ought to be played, but for one reason or another was not. To respond might be to reveal themselves in a bad light. Even among those completing the questionnaire it was often interpreted as threatening, isolating areas and activities of managerial responsibility where little was being done. An analysis of current Regional strategic plans suggests a similar general unease about the manpower component. (34)

Four questions will be discussed in this section. Firstly, what awareness was there of manpower as a resource within planning at the local level? Secondly, who was preparing the manpower input to planning, and what difficulties arose? Thirdly, how was that input drawn up, regarding both the demand and supply side? Fourthly, how did the survey respondents at the Area and District level think that manpower planning should be developed?

The awareness of manpower

Several items in the questionnaire focused on the importance attached to manpower and the awareness of manpower within the 1978/9 planning round. A majority of respondents indicated that manpower considerations were tacked on at the end once the plan was complete in its other sections. Personnel officers said that considerably greater importance was attached to the manpower input in this round compared with 1977. They were, perhaps, emphasising their own greater involvement in the planning process. One personnel officer commented, 'I was not a member of the (planning) team until late 1978. The Region sent back the (draft) plan, with the comment "add manpower" . . . Until manpower had to be done, it was not done.' However, many remarked that immediate pressures of industrial relations left personnel officers little time to devote to what was regarded as the comparatively longer term demands of manpower planning. The planners, on the other hand, saw the need for further and more detailed work in the area. They were also criticised for focusing unduly on patient flows and population issues to the detriment of manpower.

Manpower was perceived as a constraint in achieving the plan by 73 per cent of the planning officers and 82 per cent of the personnel officers. Exactly how it was a constraint varied. Manpower was seen by some as being as important as finance. For others, there was the more operational problem of the availability of staff, except that 'no real thought whatsoever has been given to whether we will be in a position to attract and keep staff during the time period'; or, the authority had experienced few recruitment problems. Indeed, if manpower was a constraint, many commented that it only affected the timescale of the implementation of the plan. As one respondent summed up the situation:

'(On the one hand) . . . manpower is a constraint . . . On the other hand, in the absence of a clear understanding by the planning mechanism of the how, whys and wherefores of manpower planning and the contribution it ought to make and can make, . . . we haven't begun yet really to do forward planning.'

This impression was further cemented by the widely held view that planners tend to be more concerned with buildings than people. 'We tend not to plan with staff in mind' was the comment of one planner, although there was a feeling that such an orientation was on the decline. This view was echoed by a personnel officer commenting that 'until recently, no great importance was attached to manpower planning.' But, commented another, 'manpower will be the key issue for a long time to come. Many users, however, still see their service aspirations met primarily with buildings, without giving detailed thought to the staffing issues related to them.' It was agreed by two out of three respondents that not enough was being done to get health service managers to 'think manpower'. 'Thinking planning', increasing the involvement of personnel in planning, together with far improved sources of information on guidelines and norms, and better training in manpower planning and its benefits were mentioned as the most likely candidates requiring action. 'Bully the planners', 'remind people of scarcities' were catchphrases thrown out. 'Attention (needs to be drawn) to the difficulty in implementing service plans without a manpower analysis, and the need to prepare training programmes.'

Such thoughts on ways forward bore close resemblance to the key issues the respondents perceived on the manpower planning side of their work. Planners tended to be more concerned with getting manpower into the plan and assessing need, while personnel officers wanted to establish the credibility of the personnel function in the whole exercise, and to generate and know how to use a valid and reliable data base on staffing. This at least squared with the frequently expressed opinion of planners that it was up to the Area and District Personnel Officers to become the 'experts' in manpower planning. In other words, planners saw their role as being one of co-ordination of the plan itself, with manpower as one input, itself co-ordinated and even generated by personnel. Manpower awareness in the sampled health authorities was therefore low, but increasing. Pressures came from two sides: the planner, wanting to get planning done properly; the personnel officer, wishing to establish credibility and keep manpower planning under his wing.

Preparation of the manpower plan

From looking at the attitude and awareness of manpower discussion moves on to explore the involvement of officers in planning, both strategic and operational, to find out what difficulties were encountered in preparing the manpower input, and to identify the perceived roles of planning and personnel officers.

The general impression was that personnel officers were peripheral to the whole exercise of preparing the relevant plan. Even where they were involved in team discussions, it was most often on the basis of providing advice or information rather than acting as full time members. One AHA officer commented that he was only brought on to the team after Region had returned the draft plan with the request 'add manpower'. This general conclusion of relative non involvement is reinforced upon examination of those actually concerned with drawing up the manpower component. In strategic planning the Area Medical Officer and the appropriate medical manpower committee, and the Area Nursing Officer or Area Nurse concerned with planning or personnel, took responsibility for their specialist groups, with the Area Medical Officer together perhaps with a specialist in Community Medicine looking after the paramedics, leaving the Area Personnel Officer to deal with clerical, ancillary and administrative staff. In only a few instances was the personnel officer drawing up the manpower plan in collaboration with the above officers and planners. Practice in operational planning was similar. In most authorities the personnel officers merely gave advice when asked. A few had co-ordinating responsibility for the whole exercise - at least where manpower planning was a formal activity. That one personnel officer should plead that he did not know 'if there is a manpower component in our plan' was far from atypical, as too were comments that no-one was preparing the manpower input.

It is hardly surprising that most respondents indicated that they had experienced difficulties in inserting a manpower input into the plans. The problems mentioned ranged very widely but most often were put down to a lack of time, expertise or interest. The initial difficulty was to get any manpower planning under way at all, with or without the co-operation of other officers. 'Limited enthusiasm on the part of senior managers in the personnel function' was one complaint. Manpower planning could hardly be attempted unless there were adequate staff resources and commitment. In addition there were considerable technical problems to be overcome, such as developing skills and producing an adequate data base. 'Information, objective criteria, and lack of knowledge - these are the problems' commented another. Given that there was an acceptance (albeit often grudging) that manpower planning had a part to play in health service management, it was unfortunate that development had not taken place because of dis-agreement and suspicion between officers from different departments and levels in the organisation as to 'who should be doing what'. 'Manpower planning within personnel: planners to liaise, work closely (with us) . . .' was a typical view presented by personnel officers. Others offered a more dynamic viewpoint, arguing that 'over optimistic assumptions regarding supply' should be challenged. Again, 'personnel (has) a crucial role, to preach, . . . (and to) lead and support line managers', or to be 'a catalyst . . . (and to provide) support and advice to service planners.' In addition, as one respondent commented, 'there is a desperate need for high quality manpower planning advice to be available for team and authority members.'

Manpower input: demand and supply

Respondents were asked to indicate the criteria used in drawing up the demand for manpower. Scanning the responses it was apparent that no or very few criteria were employed. Reference was frequently made to the utilisation of norms and guidelines, both national and Regional - usually entered where local circumstances indicated a shortfall compared with elsewhere - or to such important yet intangible (in their exact link to manpower) items as beds and workload. Equally evident were the pronouncements of selected authorities. 'What the consultants considered necessary' was the invariable solution provided for medical manpower planning, with obvious consequences for all other staff groups. There were also instances of capital led demands for staff. Demand estimates thus appeared to be based on subjective assessment with little support from quantified criteria and loosely describable as guesses; '. . . not scientific . . . (but based on)

one's own local knowledge. If medics increase the number of nurses
. . . Managers don't know the norms.' This is perhaps not surprising
in a situation where, as one respondent put it, 'we haven't got the
information to compare staffing levels. What is a right level anyway?
We need more work of a work study type to look at productivity.'

The forecasting of the supply of manpower was even more poorly thought
through or substantiated. Indeed the predominant response was that no
consideration was given to the supply side, '. . . except for nursing
staff attached for training.' It was rather expected that supply
would take care of itself. '(There is a) realisation that certain
staff groups are in short supply. That doesn't prevent people from
hoping.' A small minority gave assurances that supply was taken into
account but evidence of practical steps in this direction was difficult
to identify. Several stated that 'problem areas and shortages' were
identified, or 'developments (were) given priority according to likely
availability of staff', or 'the DMT takes this into account.' What
must be the pervasive feeling about authorities' attitudes was summed up
by one personnel officer as 'Hope, and leave personnel to find the
staff.'

If manpower planning in this round of strategic planning is demand
based - even that is an exaggeration since it is more a question of
which side, supply or demand, is ignored the most - then there is
considerable scope to greatly improve the supply forecasts. Much of
the inaction on these fronts could be explained by the felt inability of
local management to influence the situation. In response to a question
concerning their authorities' ability to influence the supply of staff,
half saw no possibilities. Others mentioned the role of training ('but
we run the risk of losing them to other AHAs'), recruitment drives,
pressures on the relevant professions, substitution of one staff group
by the less skilled, and thoughts on how to 'sell' the authority to
potential recruits. 'We have to have a sensitive network, otherwise
we won't survive' commented one officer. And '(we must) make jobs
attractive, sell the Area, accommodate career expectations, . . . (use)
intra professional word of mouth.' Even those authorities with long
standing recruitment problems presented a stoical face. It is
difficult to know whether the possible influences on supply have not
been considered at all or simply accorded to low priority.

As commentators have frequently noted the shortage of necessary
information for manpower planning in the NHS, respondents were asked
what their information base was and their interest in an information
base arising from such a system as STAMP. Most officers reported that
they had little or only very basic information on which they could draw
to prepare the manpower input. It was usually manually collected, and
stored in such a manner that even where it would have proved useful it
would have taken too long to retrieve. 'Existing staffing levels,
service needs, demands and norms', 'very basic knowledge of staff in
post', 'staffing returns from managers', were sources mentioned.
Questions were raised over the accuracy and relevance of the information
and the adequacy of current staffing levels. To say, as one personnel
officer did, that the health service was 'in the dark ages as far as
information is concerned' hardly exaggerates the feeling of his
colleagues in other authorities.

Information is thus seen as a problem area which demands quick action, although local health authorities seemed not to have thought through how such an improvement might be achieved. High hopes were being placed in STAMP. Personnel officers were better informed on its possible contribution and planners were less likely to have pressured for STAMP within the Region. This graphically illustrated where the respective officers felt that responsibility for information collection on staff and manpower planning lay. Without a manpower information system it is perhaps easier to justify the limited activity in manpower planning. However, a system such as STAMP can only facilitate the process of determining where staffing problems are likely to arise - or some of them at least. It will not provide answers to questions over the adequacy or appropriateness of staffing levels, or ensure that a more extensive and systematic consideration of supply is undertaken. In addition, as one officer commented, 'STAMP is a great improvement, but (we) still cannot analyse staff by care groups.' More fundamentally, it will not guarantee or generate a manpower plan. Perhaps it will act as an added stimulus to set the manpower planning process into operation. As one respondent commented, the information though more accessible through STAMP has always been there.

Manpower planning: the future

How do officers envisage that manpower planning needs to develop by the next round of strategic planning? The intentions of personnel to increase their role has been mentioned, as has the desire of planners to get a manpower component properly incorporated into the planning process. Equally there were hopes for an improved information base. Two further aspects were explored in the questionnaire. These centre on whether the respondent felt that the manpower input might be drawn up differently, and whether managerial ability to influence demand and supply of manpower would be increased. Nearly everyone thought that the manpower input had still to be fully accorded its proper importance. For many the advance would simply be for the manpower input to be there and not ignored. Others were able to think ahead to suggest modifications on the technical side ranging from better costings, need quantification and norms, to an earlier consideration of the manpower input and the involvement of personnel in the task. 'There should be a definitive contribution from personnel at an earlier stage in the planning process' was a frequent comment. More work on the supply side was also seen as essential. '(Better) manpower data base for forecasting . . . now we are focusing on demand. We want to shift to supply.' Many of the respondents hoped that they would be in a better position to influence the demand and supply side of manpower. 'Only the awareness throughout authorities of the importance of manpower as a resource will change the demand side of the equation. AHAs have little control on the supply side. However, they can report deficiencies through Region to a national level.' Another remarked '(I) hope I can increase my influence. I want to test it particularly with respect to supply.' The expressed hope of all was that they would have the opportunity to do a proper job on manpower 'next time round'.

THE ROLE OF THE LOCAL LEVEL

The final section of this chapter aims to throw further light on the role of the local level, of particular importance following earlier discussion over the necessity of the devolution of manpower planning responsibilities from the centre. The survey respondents were asked what role they thought the various health service tiers should play in manpower planning from DHSS to the District. Area and District officers tended to reaffirm their own level's function in manpower planning. They were rather less convinced that others were playing the correct part. They were especially critical of the role played by neighbouring tiers. They were also confirming their own formal planning role (strategic or operational).

The general view of the respondents was that the DHSS had to provide 'an overview of the national situation'. This covered activities as varied as ensuring that national supply is adequate, co-ordinating training of medics, paramedics and nurses, developing and disseminating norms and guidelines, and encouraging developments such as STAMP. For example, '(the DHSS) . . . should take action to ensure that the national supply of professional staff is adequate', or '(it) . . . should provide broad manpower guidelines/norms for action in the field.' The Region's role was similar, but with a narrower Regional perspective; it was a 'mini-DHSS'. It entailed co-ordination of manpower plans, the provision of advice to authorities, data provision, the dissemination of norms and guidelines, and medical manpower supply. While its role in medical manpower planning was widely acknowledged, this seemed to relate more to a confirmation of existing divisions of labour than a conviction that this was an optimum distribution of responsibility between tiers.

The Area officers were the most assertive that they had a key role to perform, not surprisingly given the pressures on this tier. (35) They felt that they were drawing all of the disparate pressures and interests together into a coherent plan. In this sense they were the ones 'doing the manpower planning'. Indeed their role was seen as a strategic one and as encouraging the District to undertake operational manpower planning. For example, '(the Area) . . . must identify all of their manpower demands in a strategic plan context and also . . . demonstrate how these demands may be met, including the establishment of training facilities and local policies for retention', and '. . . co-ordinate proposals from Districts and incorporate them in a priority order.' This view of the Area's role was typically rejected by the District officers. They affirmed that manpower planning had to be carried out at the District level, where the essential information on demand and supply issues was generated. The task was 'to quantify demand and inform regarding supply difficulties.' The critical role of the managerial heads in quantifying demand was also strongly emphasised. The District was thus seen as determining needs and priorities and informing others - who, and to do what, was unstated - of difficulties on the supply of staff. While Area officers held more to the formal (planning) division of responsibility, District officers were more assertive of the need for devolution.

Despite the disagreement between Areas and Districts over the exact division of responsibility, there is nothing but support for the key role that the local health authority must play in manpower planning.

Such a view was echoed in the separate responses of the Regional focal points on manpower planning, finding particular expression in the importance attached to providing advice and assistance to Areas and Districts and in discussing with them future manpower trends. These opinions tally with those who argue for the further devolution of managerial responsibilities in the health service. The impending reorganisation of the NHS which will abolish the Area tier will reinforce the (formal) role of the local (District) health authority in manpower planning, uniting in one authority both a strategic and an operational function. At the same time the Region's role will become potentially greater, embracing the area of the co-ordination of manpower planning particularly regarding training intake levels for medical and paramedical staff, that is, all staff currently trained outside the District. (36) However, it must be pointed out that at present little manpower planning is being carried out by the local health authorities. Indeed, there is a manifest lack of expertise, resources and, in some cases, interest in developing this part of the managerial role. Considerable support will be required to ensure a take off in manpower planning at this local level.

CONCLUSION

This chapter began by examining two contrasting views of manpower planning in the NHS; one arguing for the need for a central manpower planning body to cover all trained staff, the other that such a body was totally impracticable except for medical and dental staff. The devolution of manpower planning was needed, though exactly what part the various levels from DHSS to District should play was unclear. An examination of the local level in the NHS planning system and in the generation and exploration of the demand and supply of manpower, and the analysis of the survey findings on current practice of manpower planning, further illustrated the support in the NHS for devolution and helped to crystallise the role individual tiers might perform.

However, the discussion of the survey findings has shown that the innovation of manpower planning at the local level has received a less than enthusiastic reaction. Firstly, there was a limited though increasing awareness of manpower within planning. The confusion over who was to do what and the relative isolation of the personnel officer from the planning team has not helped. Secondly, the technical side of manpower planning has been slow to develop. Not only was little known about the composition of the existing workforce but little attention had been given to the future demand or supply of staff. Criteria for demand were undeveloped and minimal consideration given to supply. Some envisaged little difficulty in obtaining the manpower while others saw the impossibility of exerting influence over it either in an operational or strategic context. At the same time manpower planning tended to be interpreted as an exclusively technical exercise. The necessary conciliation and co-ordination of the respective interests on manpower appeared to have been separated from the activities of manpower planning. Thirdly, in looking forward to the next round of strategic planning, the key issue was for manpower planning to exist. It was hoped that the availability of a manpower information system such as STAMP would provide the base.

These findings lend some support to Stocking's argument concerning the pull towards centralised manpower planning in the NHS. An important task was envisaged for the centre in co-ordinating activities and in assisting in solving problems on the supply side. While the role of the local level, especially the District, was critical in relation to manpower demand, officers were commenting that they had to inform others over supply difficulties. However, such comments need to be interpreted with caution. They may reflect the limited current activity in this field, especially at the local level, rather than represent a realistic assessment of their potential. Indeed the necessity for the development of an integrated, care group approach to manpower planning, which the local level must instigate, and the exertion of influence over manpower supply (and demand), reinforce the vital role to be played at this level in the organisation. The need for a more positive approach to manpower planning, indicated by the Merrison Report, is underlined. An unintended outcome of the impending restructuring of the NHS may be to discourage the local health authority from exploring its many potential influences over the demand and supply of manpower and support a continued low level of local activity in the area of manpower planning.

Until manpower planning is incorporated and integrated into planning, whoever does it, the planner or the personnel officer, planning will not be as effective as it should be. In addition, manpower planning needs to be carried out across staff groups and not simply within them. The role of the local health authority should be both to foster an integrated approach across staff groups and to explore its influence over the demand and supply of manpower. Districts and Areas must consider how they can make best use of their present and future manpower to the benefit of their populations.

145

NOTES

(1) For example, Royal Commission on Medical Education, *Report*, (Todd Report), Cmnd. 3569, HMSO, London 1978; Committee on Nursing, *Report*, (Briggs Report), Cmnd. 5115, HMSO, London 1972; Department of Education and Science, *Speech Therapy Services*, (Quirk Report), HMSO, London 1972.

(2) The DHSS provided a useful backcloth in, 'NHS Planning: The Use of Staffing Norms and Indicators for Manpower Planning', DHSS letter from C.P.Goodale to Regional and Area administrators, April 1978.

(3) See, R.Petch, 'The Role of the DHSS', Chapter Six of this volume.

(4) For examples of Regional assistance, see the contributions in Chapter Seven of this volume.

(5) B.Stocking, 'Confusion or Control? Manpower in the Complementary Health Professions', in G.McLachlan, B.Stocking and R.F.A.Shegog (eds), *Patterns for Uncertainty? Planning for the Greater Medical Profession*, Nuffield Provincial Hospitals Trust, Oxford University Press, Oxford 1979, pp.81-136; Royal Commission on the National Health Service, *Report*, (Merrison Report), HMSO, London 1979.

(6) This is Stocking's term. She assumes that medical staff will be planned at a central (national) level, as they are at present.

(7) Stocking, 'Confusion or Control?', p.85.

(8) *Ibid.*, p.85. She concludes with the comment, 'whether the manpower planning task is carried out by central government itself or by some independent commission the DHSS and the NHS will have to play a major part.' Exactly what part the NHS would play is unspecified.

(9) *Merrison Report*, para.12.72.

(10) *Ibid.*, para.12.60.

(11) *Ibid.*, para.12.61.

(12) *Ibid.*, para.12.62.

(13) *Ibid.*, para.12.62.

(14) *Ibid.*, para.12.62.

(15) *Ibid.*, para.12.64.

(16) In the view of the Royal Commission manpower information has been a key stumbling block to manpower planning in the NHS. The SASP table on manpower is itself problematic given divergence over how to fill it in. Who was to complete the table (the Region or the Area) and on what basis (ideal or expected staffing) was unclear. Questions of accuracy and consistency are raised. Indeed there is a questionmark over whether or not all the SASP tables will be completed by Regions. See, 'Strategic Planning in 1978: Planning Manual', DHSS letter from R.S.King to Regional administrators, January 1978.

(17) Merrison Report, paras.16.61 and 12.72. See also, DHSS, *Medical Manpower - The Next Twenty Years*, HMSO, London 1978.

(18) *Merrison Report*, para.12.58.

(19) Resource Allocation Working Party (RAWP), *Sharing Resources for Health in England*, HMSO, London 1976.

(20) See, M.Blunt, 'A Case Study of Trent RHA', in Chapter Seven of this volume.

(21) This issue is explored in greater detail in Chapter Nine of this volume.

(22) See, for example, DHSS, *The Way Forward*, HMSO, London 1977; and Chapter Two of this volume.

(23) *Merrison Report*, para.12.72.

(24) *Ibid.*, para.12.72. Presumably the reference is to the DHSS's overall policy.

(25) DHSS, <u>Management Arrangements for the Reorganised National Health Service</u>, HMSO, London 1972, in such a phrase as 'maximum delegation downwards matched by accountability upwards'; DHSS, <u>Patients First</u>, HMSO, London 1979.

(26) DHSS, <u>Patients First</u>, para.5, p.2.

(27) It should be noted that the DHSS consultative document <u>Patients First</u> indicates that the present planning system will be simplified in discussion with the service (para.36).

(28) The time period of operational planning (three years) poses a problem when considering staff training as, for nearly all trained staff, at least a three year programme is required. Flexibility in interpretation is essential.

(29) DHSS, <u>Medical Manpower</u>. The Royal Commission itself says little, although there is a hint in para.12.64 (<u>Merrison Report</u>).

(30) A.Mejia, 'The Health Manpower Process', in T.L.Hall and A.Mejia (eds), <u>Health Manpower Planning</u>, World Health Organisation, Geneva 1978, p.36.

(31) Of course the biggest difficulty lies with the acute programme, accounting for around 70 per cent of expenditure within the hospital. Other definitions of programmes are possible. See, G.Mooney, 'Programme Budgetting in an Area Health Board', <u>Hospital and Health Services Review</u>, November 1977, pp.379-384; and A.Mills, 'Programme Definition and Programme Budgetting within the NHS Planning System', Nuffield Centre for Health Services Studies, University of Leeds, January 1979.

(32) See Chapter Two of this volume for a discussion of approaches to demand estimation; also, T.L.Hall, 'Supply', in Hall and Mejia, <u>Health Manpower Planning</u>.

(33) Grateful acknowledgement is made to all the respondents for their co-operation, and to the University of Leeds for financial support. The survey findings have been summarised elsewhere in, A.F.Long and G.Mercer, 'Manpower Planning in the NHS - A Report of a Survey', Nuffield Centre for Health Services Studies, University of Leeds, April 1980; and A.F.Long and G.Mercer, 'NHS Manpower Planning - Towards a Positive Approach?', <u>Health Services Manpower Review</u>, vol.6, nos.2 and 3, 1980.

(34) Strategic planning in this context covers the period 1979-1988, and operational planning 1979-1981.

(35) The survey questionnaire was sent to respondents in May/June 1979, a month or so before the Merrison Report was published.

(36) See, N.Bosanquet, 'Letter to the Editor', <u>The Guardian</u>, 17 December 1979.

9 Towards a Positive Approach
A. F. Long and G. Mercer

In this book contributors have outlined a range of perspectives on the
state of manpower planning in the NHS, providing the context within
which it takes place, indicating aspects of good practice and highlighting areas where improvements need to be made. In this chapter,
key problem areas are reviewed and possible changes examined. An
attempt is made to draw out the main themes and issues of the previous
discussion, and to explore the ways in which a more positive approach to
manpower planning can be developed in the NHS. In so doing, the role
of the local manager will be discussed. It is not implied that the
contributors to this volume adopt a common stance or are agreed about
how manpower planning in the NHS should develop. This discussion
represents the viewpoint of the editors.

THEMES AND PROBLEM AREAS

The context in which manpower operates in the NHS is the starting point.
As the pressure to increase both the level and range of health services
has intensified, the country's economic difficulties have allowed less
scope to treat sympathetically the ever rising health service bill.
The major factor in the NHS budget, manpower, is an obvious target for
expenditure cuts. Restriction of revenue threatens the quality of the
service provided to the public, as well as the financial rewards
available to, and the job commitment of, the workforce. It is against
this background that the past decade has witnessed a dramatic escalation
in industrial conflict. For its part, the Conservative Government has
taken a stand to reduce public spending, and as part of that programme
the NHS has been heavily leant upon to manage its resources more
efficiently. Previous policies to introduce a new system for the
allocation of resources, together with national guidance on priorities,
have been brought into sharper focus. Revenue, capital and manpower
have become the main targets for managerial concern. To make headway,
the health service has been taken in the direction of corporate
planning. The new system has formalised manpower planning within
health service management. The overall trend is towards the rationalisation of services and facilities.

Against this background of strict financial limits (no growth) and of

148

a new planning system, pressures to plan services and associated manpower are great. Basic problems exist though over the purpose of manpower planning and over the questions of who is to do it, how, at what level in the NHS, and with what information. Manpower planning is not however a magic wand that planning administrators can wave to suddenly make all things change. Planning the numbers and types of staff needed to provide the appropriate level of health care would be easier if staff roles were more flexible - thus allowing the substitution of one staff group by another with less or different qualifications and training - and if it was possible to determine what individual staff groups contributed to health care. Any attempt to reorientate health service staff must expect strong professional and union reaction.

Within this environment the case studies of good practice within the nursing, paramedical and medical staff groups underline the simplicity of the methodology of exploring the demand and supply positions. In McAleavey and Naylor's study the critical aspect was drawing up a realistic model of the manpower structure. Once that conceptual (and factual) task was completed, future recruitment and training needs could be estimated using available information on staff in post, and past recruitment, promotion and retirement rates. Specialist assistance was only required to transfer the manual model on to the computer in order to overcome the tedium of manual calculations. (1) Similarly, Blunt's study of occupational therapists was a survey investigation into their supply and demand. The resultant information was, however, of paramount importance for planning and policy making. In both these case studies more information was the result, presented in a more appropriate format and attempting to answer the policy question posed. In addition, the methodologies can be straightforwardly applied by the local managers, and personnel and planning officers. In contrast, Dixon developed a methodology for estimating the demand for medical manpower for use by the local officers. These three case studies, therefore, outline ways in which manpower planning practice can be developed at a local level with a minimum of specialist support. It is essential for such methodologies to be explored in manpower planning if it is to be carried out effectively and fed into the planning system.

The DHSS has an important facilitating role. It is in a pivotal position to organise developments through RAWP and to act as a political guide; its commitment to the planning system is not in doubt. However, the NHS is far from being a monolithic organisation which bows easily or quickly to central commands. Initiatives of considerable importance have been taken with the development of MIB, the broadening of MAPLIN, the encouragement and funds for the development of STAMP, and developments within the planning system itself, such as the SASP tables. However, questionmarks must be raised over the ability of the DHSS to affect the demand and supply position of staff, and thus make use of information arising from Regional strategic plans and the SASP table on manpower. Considering the supply side, once an imbalance has been identified, has the DHSS the power and the will to affect training intake levels for doctors, nurses or paramedics? And if influence was exerted, what guarantee is there that the qualifying staff would end up in places of need? The NHS has not followed the road, adopted by some other countries, of requiring so many years' service in a particular locality in return for training - one potential tactic to overcome critical local shortages of staff. Harrison's argument that manpower planning operates in a political context indicates how such issues confront more than technical barriers. Whatever the methods of estimating supply and demand, the lack of full control over such items as numbers in training or local labour markets will impress the political dimension on to manpower planning. Even in the area of information, where it has funded the development of a standardised manpower information system (STAMP), the impotence of the DHSS can be seen. The NHS demonstrates much diversity in conditions and thinking, which makes for an often uneasy relationship between centre and periphery.

The birth of STAMP has been accorded much significance. The way in which manpower information derived from STAMP can be used for manpower monitoring and manpower planning purposes is illustrated by Cree. The provision of basic information on age, length of service, turnover and costs, provides a stepping stone to begin consideration of the manpower implications and consequences of the rationalisation of services and questions of change of use. However, it must be noted that STAMP will not answer all the questions on the manpower information side. Aspects of supply fall outside of it, although indications of potential labour markets can be obtained - highlighting the need for labour market surveys as an invaluable starting point. Information cannot be equated with manpower planning. The NHS appears to have lulled itself into a sense of complacency because of the perceived promise of such an information package. In addition, the response to STAMP by NHS Regions has not been enthusiastic, ranging from jealousy to a wait-and-see attitude. Indeed, Wessex RHA itself will develop no further modules for STAMP beyond the Medical Statistics module. Yet, if STAMP succeeds in no more than encouraging a heightened awareness of manpower as a resource, a notable step forward to manpower planning will have been accomplished.

While the theory of the NHS planning system is well known, actual practice indicates that there is more lip service than enthusiasm in the adherence to corporate planning and to the manpower component within planning. Some authorities have taken significant steps towards the new system and have accorded manpower planning its intended due within their corporate approach. Elsewhere authorities perceive more pressing problems and manpower planning is barely tolerated in practice, even if sympathetic noises are made about the importance of looking at manpower in policy making. The reasons for this neglect range from direct opposition to manpower planning as an activity and a lack of expertise, to the domination of personnel's work by industrial relations matters, and to the view of planners that manpower planning is personnel's responsibility. The findings of the survey into manpower planning practice at the Region, Area and District levels highlighted these problems.

The contributions from Wessex and Trent present contrasting approaches to manpower planning within the 1978/79 strategic planning round. The relative strengths of each approach are contested within the NHS. Manpower planning and planning itself are at an early stage of application. Within Wessex the Region was playing a leading role in outlining future directions for its services, whilst Trent was summarising the Areas' intentions framed within appropriate guidelines.

Both Regions attached paramount importance to marrying manpower to available resources. Much consideration was given to the demand side, particularly through the use of service targets constrained by existing resources and translated into staff to service ratios, while very little attention was given to the supply of manpower. They also indicated the first steps towards thinking of manpower by care group, although not to planning manpower across staff groups.

The gradual establishment of the NHS planning system, and the specific pressure to fill in manpower tables as part of the strategic planning exercise for submission to the DHSS, means that manpower planning will become increasingly difficult to disregard. A more definite commitment can only be expected when there is some demonstration of the contribution which manpower planning can make to health service management. A major question at the present time revolves around the role of the different NHS authorities, particularly in the light of the likely amalgamation of authorities below Regional level. The weight of the Merrison Report was placed behind a devolution of responsibility for manpower planning, *inter alia*, to a more appropriate local level except for doctors and dentists. Unfortunately the Royal Commission report was unforthcoming on what form this might entail for manpower planning. The survey provided some helpful pointers, as too did consideration of the planning roles laid down for health authorities in the NHS planning system. DHSS was seen as playing a key co-ordinating role, concerning itself with questions of national supply, an overview of training intakes for trained staff, the development of reliable norms, the initiation of research, and the provision of a central core of expertise in manpower planning. The Region's role was similar, being that of a DHSS in miniature, while in addition having to be concerned with the development of the manpower input to Regional strategic planning. It was at the District level that manpower planning was actually seen as taking place in terms of quantifying demand and informing on questions of supply. The Area's role, while clearly perceived, appeared to be one resulting not from necessity but rather from its position in the organisational structure and its role in the planning system - providing information to Districts, encouraging manpower planning, and co-ordinating activities in a multi District situation.

To push manpower planning in its entirety to the local level, while containing many advantages, will also have its problems. The organisation of many professional associations on a national level makes for difficulties when a single local health authority wants to sort out its own problems of recruitment in a particular sector. In addition, there is the limited nature of current manpower planning at the local level. Other pressures have entered in such as industrial relations, or it has just been ignored. Manpower planning will not necessarily prosper in a wholesale delegation of responsibilities to the local level, while at the same time it is at this level, of departmental heads, that the foundations for manpower planning need to be laid.

THE CURRENT STATE OF MANPOWER PLANNING

Manpower planning in the NHS is in its infancy. For the greater part of health service managers manpower planning is poorly understood, imperfectly executed or, all too often, simply ignored. Yet there is another side to NHS manpower planning which is increasingly sophisticated in its approach and more earnest in its desire to establish manpower planning as a key element in health service policy making. With firm and increased recognition by the DHSS and the Royal Commission on the NHS the prospects for manpower planning to take off at a Regional and sub-Regional level have never been more auspicious.

At a national level, through developments such as MAPLIN and MIB, encouragement is being given to manpower planning at the Region. The emphasis has been on identifying and developing manpower planning focal points to facilitate information exchange and to provide support for manpower planning and technical advice within the Region. Following the Royal Commission's comments on devolution this emphasis is likely to be confirmed. Some Regions have developed strong manpower planning units, seeing their own role as developing manpower planning practice and expertise within the Region. Activities range from exploring manpower issues for particular staff groups to linking manpower into strategic planning and setting up training and education in manpower planning.

Moving on to the Area and District level, one can see the fundamental problems implicit in current manpower planning practice in the NHS. A limited awareness of manpower as a resource, unsystematic assessments of demand, limited information and time devoted to the subject, a lack of focus on the supply of staff, a limited involvement of personnel in planning, and confusion over who is doing the manpower planning - and so the list could continue. In sum, there is little co-ordinated manpower planning taking place.

The problems of manpower planning are far from solely organisational in origin. The technical expertise to do manpower planning has been slow to develop in the health service. Not only is little known about the make-up of the existing workforce, but little attention has been given to future problems of demand or supply. The lack of an adequate information base has been blamed as a considerable handicap to manpower planning. The demand side of manpower has tended to be taken as given, or set by revenue constraints translated into staff and services. The difficulties of assessing demand, as well as the potential for professional rivalries to be set alight, have encouraged inaction. This is an area where central initiatives, such as RAWP, have stimulated the redistribution of medical resources and thus other resources between Regions. Overall, manpower has received increased attention as a result of the need to fill in the SASP table on manpower. But much of the thinking has neglected to determine what level of staff might actually be recruited, rather than what is wanted.

Another important omission is the failure to consider alternative mixes of staff. The burden of high manpower costs together with some shortages of trained staff has encouraged a trend towards the higher utilisation of untrained staff. Little has been done to consider the wider ramifications of this development on service care. Equally, the recommendation to make staff roles more flexible and to encourage substitution across staff groups has made little progress. Finally, the vexed question of productivity is all but ignored for groups other than ancillary staff. The political nature of manpower planning is clearly to the fore.

THE LOCAL MANAGER AND MANPOWER PLANNING

Manpower planning is the job of every manager or departmental head.
The objectives are fairly specific: to maintain a reasonable level of
staffing and staffing mix whilst ensuring manpower matches available
revenue.   In other words, the manager's basic concern must be with the
maintenance of the existing workforce within the context of desired
standards of service.   As one part of this concern, and likely to be of
a lower order of priority, the manager is concerned with questions of
strategic planning and operational (manpower) implications.   The
operational aspects are well to the fore: to maintain and improve
productivity; to recruit to replace; and to contain sickness, absence
and departures.   Indeed, it is in these areas that the techniques of
manpower planning outlined in Chapter Three of this volume can be
applied with value.   For example, Blunt's exploration of the demand and
supply position of a staff group is a prerequisite to drawing up
reasonable and coherent plans.   Similarly, the methodology of McAleavey
and Naylor's study can be used by the local manager to examine recruitment and training needs.   The essential first step is the
identification of the manpower structure within the location.

If the manager's job is to maintain the workforce, what role has
personnel to play?   Information provision on manpower and norms, and
co-ordination of activities in a strategic planning context are two
possible aspects of the personnel role.   There is also the issue of who
will be taking a broader and longer term look at the workforce, and
raise questions over training intake needs.   Is the manager able to
carry this through or does personnel have a joint role to play?   The
training implications must be picked up and pressure exerted on to the
training bodies.   It is essential that the manpower input is linked
into planning.

The involvement of the local manager in planning (be it the
consultant, head of occupational therapy, or nurse manager) centres
around the maintenance, and/or improvement, of the service to be
provided to the patients.   Once the service objectives and targets
have been drawn up detailed attention needs to be given to estimating
manpower requirements and potential supply.   For the former, norms and
guidelines tend to play a critical role.   However, while they are easy
to use and interpret to others and pose minimal data demands, their use
should be restricted to providing baseline projections of numbers
required to maintain the current standard of service.   For they
encourage the neglect of the potential for improving the productivity,
distribution and utilisation of staff, and of the very relevance of the
services themselves.   Time would be better spent exploring the
dynamics and determinants of demand, and in examining the areas of
productivity, utilisation, and staffing ratios themselves, in order to
generate the most appropriate range of services for the population and
mixes of staff to provide them. (2)

The local manager, personnel and planning officers are not totally
free agents in this process of estimating manpower demands.   They are
working within a set of external induced constraints, ranging from

directives (such as the EEC directives on nurse training) and norms and guidelines (from the DHSS and the Region on service priorities and manpower ratios), to professional standards (over minimum staffing levels and ratios of trained to untrained staff) and nationally agreed pay and conditions of service (resulting in a higher cost of current staffing levels), to discretion by a higher tier whether an additional medical post can be created, and to such factors as the limited finance available, previous capital developments, available technology, and existing staff, both levels, quality and relationships. While national, Regional and professional guidelines and directives affect manpower requirements, they are open to interpretation to fit the local situation. At the local level the focus is upon the interface of the patient and the health practitioner. In addition, local pressures may arise from pressure groups such as the local Community Health Council and from interests inside the service such as one of the health professions or trade unions or other departmental heads and clinicians. For example, the consultant's desires to develop a particular service will have implications not only for the medical staff but also for nursing and other supporting staff groups right down to the level of the porters. This highlights the need for an intraprofessional, integrated approach to manpower planning across staff groups. Policies of the local manager concerning the productivity of staff and substitution of a lesser trained individual to take over the less skilled tasks of a higher trained person may be severely constrained by local trade union pressure and professional rivalries. (3)

While the estimation of manpower demands is fraught with political constraints and technical difficulties, the exploration of likely supply is similarly problematic but has greater scope for an active role to be played by managers, personnel and planning officers at the local health authority level. However, health service managers are very sceptical about the possibility of any influence over the supply of staff, except perhaps in the area of nurse training, as the survey data reported in Chapter Eight showed. Through exploring potential influences over the supply of medical and dental staff, a group for whom common opinion asserts that only the DHSS (in consultation with others, especially the BMA) can effectively operate, some of the varieties of influence open to local managers, personnel and planning officers will be raised. In this area there are currently shortages of medical staff in particular specialties (anaesthesia, geriatrics), locations, and disparities across Regions and Areas (using doctor/population ratios as a guide). Focusing on one aspect of this picture, the perceived shortage of medical staff in a local health authority (a District, Area, or new District Health Authority), what influences can be exerted to improve the supply position?

As a first step, the local health authority must investigate why it is experiencing difficulties in recruiting and/or retaining medical staff. Problems could have arisen from a lack of revenue, poor physical facilities, housing difficulties, the general attractiveness of the locality, or local personalities, to name but a few possibilities. The local health authority can therefore plan to affect the physical facilities, attempt to sell the locality to potential recruits, explore other sources of supply (that is, from the 'pool'), and alter the available posts both in terms of hours and the type of work to make them more attractive. More flexible part time contracts and the provision

of creche facilities can be provided to encourage women to continue
health services employment.   Contact can also be increased with the
profession itself and particularly with the medical schools, encouraging
attachments to the local authority, with the hope of the word spreading
that it is not such a bad place to work in after all.   The possibility
of substituting non medical personnel (for example, dental auxiliaries)
may be considered, or of expanding the duties of trained staff (for
example, to develop the role of nurse practitioner). (4)   Finally, the
local health authority can explore the productivity of its staff, and
ways of increasing it, although there are likely to be blocks to
implementation.   In a no or limited growth situation such an approach,
while unpopular with staff, assumes greater significance and
importance. (5)   It is only for training and pay and conditions of
service that the local authority cannot directly intervene to affect its
supply of medical staff.   It can only pressure the higher tiers and the
profession.   Indeed, without resort to the direction of labour (for
newly trained staff), there would be no guarantee that influences on
intake size and pay levels would result in students upon completing
their training coming to work in the locality.

Under the current structure of the NHS the Area tier has two specific
avenues of influence: over financial allocations to Districts (in a
multi District context); and discretion over a new medical post.   It
can allocate additional revenues to the District to allow expansion and
updating of physical facilities.   It can also restrict medical posts
within the other Districts in the AHA.   All the 'new' medical posts can
be given to the shortage District.   In the restructured NHS, with the
abolition of the Area tier, such possible manipulative influences will
come under the aegis of the Region.   Potential influences open to this
level shift to include the Region's medical school.   It can pressure
the DHSS and the medical school concerned to increase student intakes.
(6)   It can also, through the so called 'matching scheme', guaranteeing
employment to graduates of medical schools, change contracts of
employment to commit the newly qualified graduate to a period of
service in a 'deprived' local health authority.   In addition the
Region has, both at present and likely to be reinforced upon the
restructure of the NHS, discretion over new medical posts desired by
authorities within the Region, and it may decide to withhold approval
and finance for a particular post.   Overall, its influence is of a
different order of magnitude to that of the local authority.   The focus
is upon pressuring for increases in training numbers or in directing
staff to work in particular localities and specialties.

The recent Conservative proposals for the restructuring of the NHS and
particularly for the abolition of the Area tier further complicate the
picture of the potential influences open to authorities over the supply
of medical manpower. (7)   The Area's powers are likely to return to the
Regional level through the allocation of resources and discretion over
new posts.   However, according to the consultative document *Patients
First*, the new District Health Authorities will have responsibility for
consultant contracts (and contracts of all other staff who work in the
authority) while recognising the need for a strong advisory role at the
Regional level. (8)   As one commentator sees it, this former proposal
will make little difference to the present power of the Region '. . . as
it would soon become apparent that the final say on the creation of
consultant appointments could not be left to the districts.' (9)

Looking more broadly at the supply of manpower, the issue of determining intake levels to training schools and their co-ordination is raised. Potentially again the Region's role is being strengthened. Its '. . . informal power will be further reinforced because the new district authorities will be too small to plan many types of service or professional manpower.' (10) Notwithstanding, the local health authority will have many avenues to explore and experiment with over the supply of medical staff, and more so for other staff groups, excepting perhaps those trained outside it.

Finally, there is the role of the DHSS. It is at a national level that salary levels are fixed and decisions regarding student intake numbers for medical and dental schools made, in consultation with the profession, Regions, and the universities themselves. Accordingly, its influence on the supply of medical and dental staff within a particular District is of a remote nature. There is no clear connection between such national decisions regarding pay and student intakes and the local difficulties in a health authority. However, the DHSS can have specific influences on two fronts. Firstly, it could develop special allowances to encourage staff to work in a 'deprived', 'under-doctored' local authority on the lines of current general practitioner inducements. In other words, it can modify nationally agreed salary levels to build in the notion of local scales and allowances. Secondly, it can and does encourage medical and dental expansion within particular specialties, for example, through circulars on manpower approval for medical posts. (11)

The DHSS and the Region, therefore, have very different avenues to explore than the local health authority. Their influences lie mainly in the area of affecting student intakes, and encouraging (or restricting) medical posts in particular specialties. The DHSS could provide further assistance locally by modifying present pay procedures to allow for additional scales and allowances, and the Region through adopting a more interventionist policy on the direction of (newly trained) labour. The local health authority, on the other hand, has to be more concerned with exploring alternative sources of supply, ways of retaining and maintaining contact with staff, and means of increasing the attractiveness of the locality, ranging from updating the facilities to developing communication with the professions and the training schools. Table 9.1 (see p.157) attempts to generalise the previous discussion, and outlines the potential influences open to the local health authority, the Region, and the DHSS on the supply of manpower. The exact influences available to the authorities will vary according to the staff group in question. For example, nurse training schools are currently situated within Area authorities and service the appropriate Districts, while for paramedical groups training schools tend to be in terms of one per Region. The possibility of the local health authority to direct newly qualified staff to areas of need should not be ruled out. The above discussion concerning medical supply influences should therefore be interpreted broadly and replayed for the various staff groups and parts of them; for occupational therapists, radiographers, qualified nurses, unqualified nurses and so on.

The essential conclusion of this discussion is that there are many means of affecting the supply of manpower at each level in the NHS, particularly so at the local level, and not all concentrated at one

Table 9.1

Some Influences over the Supply of Manpower

Local Health Authority	Region	DHSS
Investigate the reason for the perceived shortage of staff or difficulties in recruitment	Alter financial allocations	Alter pay and conditions of service, and allow introduction of local scales and allowances
Improve the working environment	Influence training schools, training bodies and the DHSS	Influence training bodies
Improve staff accommodation and facilities	Direct (newly qualified) staff to designated places	Develop career structure
Mount a publicity campaign to 'sell' the locality		
Modify the hours and type of work; encourage flexibility; increase fringe benefits		
Provide creche facilities		
Explore underutilised sources of supply from the labour pool; 'nurse banks'; in-service and training courses		
Develop and increase contacts with the profession and training schools		
Assess staff productivity		
Explore substitution and role enlargement possibilities		
Direct (newly qualified) staff to designated places		

157

level. While the specific set of influences the various tiers in the organisation can exert over supply will vary for the many staff groups, no one authority has a monopoly over them. Each has a role to play, especially given the variety of labour markets for grades within a staff group and the differing locations of the training schools. The task of the local health authority and thus of the local officers, in relation to manpower demand, supply and manpower studies, needs to be underlined. They must not shirk their responsibilities, but rather explore and experiment to extend their capabilities in this area. They must test out their power, both formal and informal, of especial importance in view of the changing balance of power between the DHSS, the Region and the new District Health Authorities.

THE FUTURE OF MANPOWER PLANNING IN THE NHS

Attention finally turns to the directions along which manpower planning needs to develop in the future. As some of the contributions to this volume have shown, the 1978/79 round of strategic planning consisted at most of a stock taking exercise on existing manpower and produced solely demand based statements about manpower. Demand, while imperfectly investigated, was not as poorly treated as the supply of labour. By the next round (1982/83) considerations will have to extend to embrace both demand and supply. Accordingly, what specific organisational, political and technical developments need to be fostered to engender a more positive approach to manpower planning?

The starting point is to ask who should be doing manpower planning. The key role of the local managers, personnel and planning officers has already been stressed, particularly concerning the generation of demand and influences over the supply of manpower. Indeed, they provide the base for the whole process, in managing their own manpower, planning future requirements, and trying to ensure requisite supply is achieved. At yet another level there is the issue of the role of the Regional focal points on manpower planning. They have expended time and energy on developing the manpower information side to the detriment of questions of manpower planning as a whole, whilst Wessex as centre of responsibility was developing a national standard approach (STAMP). Such a focus is not surprising, given the lack of information in the area and the low support, if any, given to focal points in their Regions and especially by the Regional Personnel Officers. A concern with increasing the awareness of manpower as a resource through mounting reports on the demand and supply picture in a staff or client group would appear an obvious angle to pursue. In other words, energies would be better focused on showing what can be done, and establishing the credibility and value of manpower planning.

The second basic question requiring consideration is that of how manpower planning should be carried out. Manpower must be treated as a critical resource and be brought into focus within planning, and not left outside it. It is here that the role of MAPLIN must be questioned. While it is no doubt the case that MAPLIN has increased expertise in manpower planning, at the least amongst the focal points, and is very valuable as a means of interchanging information, methodology and ideas, its very existence in its present form can be seen as leading potentially to one unwelcome development: the development of manpower planning separately from planning and as a specialist area. Even though MAPLIN has a steering group of a 'national regional team of officers', the focal points themselves are predominantly from the personnel function, itself poorly integrated with planning administrators and looking to find its own role in (manpower) planning. Manpower planning is not a specialist area. It is part of every manager's job. The role of focal points must be carefully practised, not as a separate entity apart from planning, but rather from an integration with planning, and in providing expertise to assist managers and personnel to develop the manpower input to planning.

Another part of the 'how' question concerns the way the manpower input is developed. Looking firstly at the demand and supply for manpower, a more systematic approach is called for. On the demand side, the predominance of the manpower to population ratio method for demand estimation must be examined to see its appropriateness across localities. Whilst this method is easy to use, it provides little insight into how demands for manpower are generated and determined, and it encourages the neglect of the potential for improving productivity and utilisation of manpower, two areas ignored for staff groups in the NHS apart from ancillary staff. A more positive approach is to examine health needs, itself clearly delineating how and why manpower demands are generated. Secondly, to consider supply would be a step forward on the present situation. Potential influences of authorities over the supply of staff must be explored and exercised. Questions of wider employment and demographic trends also need to be examined. For example, how will current trends in educational qualifications of school leavers affect training school intakes, and similarly changes in childbearing patterns affect intake levels and staff turnover generally? (12) Indeed in some localities reductions in staffing will require attention.

Turning to the information side of manpower planning, the availability of main STAMP in 1980 will provide a common data base, common definitions and, in the longer term, provide historical data and enable comparative analyses (for example, between authorities) to be undertaken. Terminals connected to a central computer system or locally based microprocessors will be needed to ensure an immediate access to the data base and to allow prompt retrieval of ad hoc information requests. STAMP can best be described as an aid to manpower planning, in encouraging the examination of the manpower implications of policies and in increasing awareness of manpower as a resource. The gaps remaining in manpower information, particularly on the supply side, including the absence of labour market surveys, cannot be ignored.

A final issue under the question of how manpower planning in the NHS needs to develop concerns the whole approach to manpower planning itself. Adequate manpower planning is more than each head of department setting out the demands and supply position of the manpower in that staff group. It is essential that manpower planning across staff groups and not just within staff groups is fostered. Such an integrated approach to manpower planning ties into the planning system's focus on care groups while it involves more than looking at manpower by care group. On the one hand, a natural offshoot of the health care planning team approach, in a situation of awareness of manpower, would be for manpower objectives to be set within the team, indicating a range of skills required to meet the service objectives for the care group, and possible ways of achieving them. On the other hand, given the department head's objective of maintaining the workforce, if, for example, the nursing manager meets this objective, how certain is it that other staff groups will do likewise; and if they do not, what are the implications for the health care manpower team who provide a service to the patient? This leads discussion into difficult waters, encouraging professional groups to interact over the sensitive question of job content. Such discussions need to extend to questions of roles, flexibility within a role, and possibilities of substitution of the lesser qualified for the more qualified in situations of scarcity of resources, either for finance or of manpower, and productivity itself. Of course, substitution of staff already takes place in the NHS. For example, at times nurses and physiotherapists perform similar tasks. The basic objective of health care must not be forgotten: to determine the most appropriate range of services and mixes of staff to meet the patient's or care group's needs.

The third question to consider is where manpower planning should be undertaken in the NHS structure. While it should be carried out at all levels in the NHS, some activities have to be undertaken at a particular level. For example, the role of the Region should be one of co-ordination and monitoring, with the Regional focal points providing advice and expertise to assist local manpower planning. In contrast, a key activity at the local level should comprise demand generation in an integrated manner with planning. It is, therefore, important to encourage the exploration of influences over both the demand and supply of manpower at this point in the organisation and to develop local commitment. Exactly which officers should co-ordinate the activity is not as important as everyone knowing how responsibility is distributed and making sure the job gets done. The personnel officer's involvement in industrial relations need not overshadow the broader role of encouraging manpower planning by functional managers and heads of department.

The indications on the restructuring of the NHS outlined in the consultative document *Patients First* lend further support for the need to develop local expertise. While it is likely that one consequence of the abolition of the Area tier will be a strengthened role of the Region in manpower planning - in terms of the need for co-ordination over training intake levels, with the possible exception of nursing - the role of the future District Authority will be heightened with the likely addition of a strategic planning role. An unfortunate consequence might be to discourage Districts from exploring and exercising influences over the supply of manpower, placing on to the Region the responsibility of ensuring adequate local labour supply, especially if the Region were to adopt a policy of training for self-sufficiency in training capacity. Indeed, if a District is generally a net importer of newly qualified staff, perhaps it should compensate the exporting authority by paying for the training of its recruits.

A more positive approach to manpower planning must then be concerned with raising the consciousness of manpower as a prime resource, not to be wasted and ignored but encouraged to show its full potential in contributing to patient care. 'More action and less talk' would be a suitable aphorism to describe the way forward for manpower planning in the NHS. Lip service without enthusiasm needs to be turned into commitment to exploring the manpower aspects of proposals and modifying such plans if necessary. The development of local commitment and expertise, and the exploration of potential influences over supply, must occur. Without adequate manpower consideration planning is nonsensical.

All of the above areas if developed would lead to manpower in the NHS having a very different character. A commitment to think manpower (planning); service (and capital) plans incorporating manpower demand and supply considerations, by care group and across staff group while ensuring manpower matches available revenue; systematic demand estimation; an active and influential local health authority exploring and keeping in touch with supply issues; exploration of the utilisation of manpower and the potential for higher productivity; flexibility over roles; examination of how each staff group contributes to patient care. This is not a utopia, but rather the conditions for effective manpower planning in the health service.

Manpower planning in the future might with benefit be established in the following form. The health planning team having considered the needs of the care group outlines its service objectives and translates these into manpower and other objectives, ensuring finance is not exceeded. The manpower objectives indicate the range of skills required and likely implications for types of staff. The departmental manager, either as a member of the team or as a source of advice, examines the manpower objectives, exploring the needs for manpower in the department to provide the required service, including better utilisation and productivity and investigating the likely source of supply of such staff. Personnel's role in this activity is one of providing information and co-ordinating the manpower planning activity.

Many areas require further research and development. There is the dispute about whether the political dimension in planning can become more akin to a technical issue, or whether bargaining and negotiation are inherent in planning and thus manpower planning. An examination of whether and how local health authorities can exercise influence over the supply side of manpower is required. There is too the need for research into how manpower planning across staff groups can become a reality, bridging political and professional questions of role definition and demarcation. Indeed, it remains to be demonstrated whether the process of operational planning currently taking place will force the manpower aspects to the fore and spark off a heightened commitment to consider the manpower resource, not at the end but in the development of the plans themselves.

The integration of the manpower component into planning will bring into sharper focus the associated political problems of health policy formulation and its implementation. It must not be forgotten, however, that manpower planning will not eliminate all the difficulties in the planning and organisation of health service staff. There will remain unplanned and uncontrollable dimensions. Financial restraints, modifications of health treatments and health demands, the implementation of pay settlements, decisions over staff training, and shortages of labour supply - all can nullify the best laid plan. This should not provide a justification for withdrawing from manpower planning. Much of practical benefit can and should be developed as a matter of urgency.

Manpower planning in the NHS is at a basic level. Its evolution and development is unlikely to take just one form; it will not, given current approaches to planning. Commitment and expertise are spreading through the health service. However, good practice of manpower planning is hard to identify. What does it mean for a 'manpower' plan to succeed? That supply met demand, or that individual career developments tallied with service requirements, or what? Like its planning parent, planning manpower is a way of thinking, of exploring possibilities, to try to ensure the achievement of a desired future. Manpower planning must not become an end in itself. It is only a tool to assist in the process of providing appropriate health care to patients.

NOTES

(1) Computer modelling only provides a speedy analysis of the problem which could be generated manually.   The manager needs to determine when to call in the expert.

(2) See Chapters Two, Three and Seven of this volume; also, T.L.Hall, 'Demand', in T.L.Hall and A.Mejia (eds), Health Manpower Planning, World Health Organisation, Geneva 1978, pp.82-83, Table 4.

(3) For a discussion of some of these factors see, S.Harrison, 'The Politics of Health Manpower', Chapter Five of this volume.

(4) Looking at staffing figures by staff group within or between Regions, there is evidence that substitution already occurs in the NHS: for example, a smaller percentage of doctors is compensated for by a higher proportion of nurses.   For discussion of the issues of role enlargement and substitution see, R.Austin, 'Practising Health Care: The Nurse Practitioner', in P.Atkinson, R.Dingwall and A.Murcott (eds), Prospects for the National Health Service, Croom Helm, London 1979; and B.L.E.C.Reedy, 'Substitution and the Manpower Dilemma', in G.McLachlan, B.Stocking and R.F.A.Shegog (eds), Patterns for Uncertainty? Planning for the Greater Medical Profession, Nuffield Provincial Hospitals Trust, Oxford University Press, Oxford 1979.

(5) For example, see J.D.Baker, 'Productivity', in T.L.Hall and A.Mejia (eds), Health Manpower Planning; and S.R.Engleman, 'External Economic Influences on NHS Manpower', in G.McLachlan et al. (eds), Patterns for Uncertainty?.

(6) The level of student intakes is not the sole problem.   Other questions need to be raised: for example, how significant are the pool and immigration as sources of supply?   Is the Region training for its own needs or others as well?

(7) As outlined in, DHSS, 'Health Service Development: Structure and Management', DHSS Circular HC(80)8, July 1980.

(8) DHSS, Patients First, HMSO, London 1979, para.21.

(9) N.Bosanquet, 'Letter to the Editor', The Guardian, 17 December 1979.

(10) Ibid.   Indeed, this lends support to Stocking's argument for centralised manpower planning, outlined in Chapter Eight of this volume.

(11) See, DHSS, 'Medical and Dental Manpower: 1979 Specialty Review', DHSS letter to Regional administrators, 30 March 1979.

(12) See, for example, Department of Employment, 'Changing Composition of the Labour Force 1976-1991', Department of Employment Gazette, June 1979, pp.546-551.

Bibliography

Atkinson, P., Dingwall, R. and Murcott, A., Prospects for the National Health Service, Croom Helm, London 1979.

Austin, R., 'Practising Health Care: The Nurse Practitioner', in Atkinson, P., Dingwall, R. and Murcott, A. (eds), Prospects for the National Health Service, Croom Helm, London 1979, pp.145-158.

Bacon, R. and Eltis, W., Britain's Economic Problem: Too Few Producers, Macmillan, London 1976.

Baker, T., 'Productivity', in Hall, T.L. and Mejia, A. (eds), Health Manpower Planning: Principles, Methods, Issues, World Health Organisation, Geneva 1978, pp.117-132.

Barnard, K.A. and Lee, K. (eds), Conflicts in the National Health Service, Croom Helm, London 1977.

Blaug, M., 'The Uses and Abuses of Manpower Planning', New Society, 31 July 1975, pp.247-248.

Bosanquet, N., 'Letter to the Editor', The Guardian, 17 December 1979.

Brown, R., 'Structure and Local Policy Making in the Making of the Reorganised National Health Service', Public Administration Bulletin, no.20, 1976, pp.9-19.

Cambridge Area Health Authority (Teaching), A Computerised Manpower Information System, King's Fund Project Paper, London 1976.

Central Statistical Office, Annual Abstract of Statistics, HMSO, London 1955.

Central Statistical Office, Annual Abstract of Statistics, HMSO, London 1978.

Child, J. (ed.), Man and Organisation, Allen and Unwin, London 1973.

Civil Service Department, A Management Guide to Manpower Planning Models, HMSO, London 1975.

Clegg, H.A. and Chester, T.E., Wage Policy and the Health Services, Blackwell, Oxford 1957.

Clode, D., 'Circling the Pyramid by Camel - via the Needle's Eye', Health and Social Services Journal, 3 August 1979, pp.972-975.

Committee of Enquiry into Mental Handicapped Nursing and Care, Report, (Jay Report), Cmnd. 7468, HMSO, London 1979.

Committee of Enquiry into the Cost of the National Health Service, Report, (Guillebaud Report), Cmnd. 9663, HMSO, London 1956.

Committee of Enquiry into the Pay and Related Conditions of Service of the Professions Supplementary to Medicine and Speech Therapists, Report, (Halsbury Report), HMSO, London 1975.

Committee on Local Authority and Allied Services, Report, (Seebohm Report), HMSO, London 1968.

Committee on Nursing, Report, (Briggs Report), Cmnd. 5115, HMSO, London 1972.

Committee on the Senior Nursing Structure, Report, (Salmon Report), HMSO, London 1966.

Committee to Consider the Future Numbers of Medical Practitioners and the Appropriate Intake of Medical Students, Report, (Willink Report), HMSO, London 1957.

Council for Professions Supplementary to Medicine, Annual Report 1977/78, London 1978.

Crick, B., In Defence of Politics, Pelican, Harmondsworth 1964.

Dearden, R., 'Why the Planning System is a Good Thing Provided We Don't

Stick to the Rules', Hospital and Health Services Review, October 1978, pp.345-346.

Department of Education and Science, Speech Therapy Services, (Quirk Report), HMSO, London 1972.

Department of Employment, Company Manpower Planning, HMSO, London 1968.

Department of Employment, 'Changing Composition of the Labour Force 1976-1991', Department of Employment Gazette, June 1979.

Department of Employment, Disclosure of Information to Trade Unions for Collective Bargaining Purposes, Code of Practice no.2, HMSO, London 1977.

Department of Employment, Employment Protection Act 1975, HMSO, London 1975.

Department of Employment, Health and Safety at Work Act 1974, HMSO, London 1974.

DHSS, 'Closure or Change of Use of Health Buildings', DHSS Circular HSC(IS)207, 1975.

DHSS, Absence from Work, DHSS, London 1975.

DHSS, 'Health Service Development: Structure and Management', DHSS Circular HC(80)8, July 1980.

DHSS, 'Health Service Planning in England 1976-1978', DHSS, London 1979.

DHSS, Leavers (Standard Measures and Classifications), DHSS, London 1975.

DHSS, Management Arrangements for the Reorganised National Health Service, HMSO, London 1972.

DHSS, 'Medical and Dental Manpower: 1979 Specialty Review', DHSS letter to Regional administrators, 30 March 1979.

DHSS, Medical Manpower - The Next Twenty Years, A Discussion Paper, HMSO, London 1978.

DHSS, National Health Service Reorganisation: England, Cmnd. 5055, HMSO, London 1972.

DHSS, 'NHS Planning: The Use of Staffing Norms and Indicators for Manpower Planning', DHSS letter from C.P. Goodale to Regional and Area administrators, April 1978.

DHSS, Operation and Development of Services: Organisation for Personnel Management, NHS Reorganisation Circular HRC(73)37, 1973.

DHSS, Patients First, HMSO, London 1979.

DHSS, 'Planning Guidelines for 1978-79', DHSS Circular HC(78)12, 1978.

DHSS, 'Planning Guidelines for 1979-80', DHSS Circular HC(79)9, 1979.

DHSS, Priorities for Health and Personal Social Services in England, HMSO, London 1976.

DHSS, 'Qualifications', MAPLIN Report no.3, 1979.

DHSS, 'Strategic Planning in 1978: Planning Manual', DHSS letter from R.S. King to Regional administrators, January 1978.

DHSS, Staffing of the National Health Service (England): An Analysis of the Demand and Supply Positions in the Major Staff Groups, DHSS, London 1979.

DHSS, The NHS Planning System, HC(76)30, DHSS, London 1976.

DHSS, Recruitment and Training of Dental Hygienists, (Interim Report), HMSO, London 1974.

DHSS, The Way Forward, HMSO, London 1977.

Donald, B.L., Manpower for Hospitals, Institute of Hospital Administrators, London 1966.

Donald, B.L., 'Towards a More Positive Manpower Policy', Health Services Manpower Review, vol.3, no.3, 1977.

Eckstein, H., The English Health Service, Harvard University Press, Massachusetts 1970.

Engleman, S.R., 'External Economic Influences on NHS Manpower', in McLachlan, G., Stocking, B. and Shegog, R.F.A. (eds), Patterns for Uncertainty? Planning for the Greater Medical Profession, Nuffield Provincial Hospitals Trust, Oxford University Press, Oxford 1979, pp.165-184.

Flanders, A., Management and Unions: The Theory and Reform of Industrial Relations, Faber, London 1970.

Fox, A., 'Industrial Relations: A Social Critique of Pluralist Ideology', in Child, J. (ed.), Man and Organisation, Allen and Unwin, London 1973, pp.185-233.

Gough, I., 'State Expenditure in Advanced Capitalism', New Left Review, no.92, 1975, pp.53-92.

Gough, I., The Political Economy of the Welfare State, Macmillan, London 1979.

Gray, D.H., Manpower Planning, Institute of Personnel Management, London 1976.

Gunn, L. and Mair, R., 'Staffing the National Health Service', in McLachlan, G. (ed.), Challenges for Change, Nuffield Provincial Hospitals Trust, Oxford University Press, Oxford 1971, pp.263-295.

Hall, T.L., 'Demand', in Hall, T.L. and Mejia, A. (eds), Health Manpower Planning: Principles, Methods, Issues, World Health Organisation, Geneva 1978, pp.57-90.

Hall, T.L., 'Supply', in Hall, T.L. and Mejia, A. (eds), Health Manpower Planning: Principles, Methods, Issues, World Health Organisation, Geneva 1978, pp.91-116.

Hall, T.L. and Kleczkowski, M., 'Manpower Planning and the Political Process', in Hall, T.L. and Mejia, A. (eds), Health Manpower Planning: Principles, Methods, Issues, World Health Organisation, Geneva 1978, pp.299-331.

Hall, T.L. and Mejia, A. (eds), Health Manpower Planning: Principles, Methods, Issues, World Health Organisation, Geneva 1978.

Ham, C.J., 'Power, Patients and Pluralism', in Barnard, K.A. and Lee, K. (eds), Conflicts in the National Health Service, Croom Helm, London 1977, pp.99-120.

Hart, J.T., 'The Inverse Care Law', Lancet, vol.1, 1971.

Health Services Organisation Research Unit, Brunel University, 'Organisation of Physiotherapy and Occupational Therapy in the NHS', Working Paper, 1977.

House of Commons Expenditure Committee, Eleventh Report, vol.II, pt.1, HMSO, London 1977.

Hussey, D., Corporate Planning: Theory and Practice, Pergamon, Oxford 1974.

Hyman, R. and Brough, I., Social Values and Industrial Relations, Blackwell, Oxford 1975.

Joint Working Party on the Medical Staffing Structure in the Hospital Service, Report, (Platt Report), HMSO, London 1961.

Klein, R.E., 'Policy Options for Medical Manpower', British Medical Journal, 19 July 1979.

Kogan, M., The Working of the National Health Service, Royal Commission on the National Health Service, Research Paper no.1, HMSO, London 1978.

Körner, E., 'The Importance of Being Earnest about Planning', Hospital and Health Services Review, October 1979.

Levitt, R., The Reorganised National Health Service, Croom Helm, London 1976.

Lewin, D., 'An Approach to Area Strategic Planning: Report for the

Operational Research Service of the DHSS', February 1979.

Lind, G., Luckman, J. and Wiseman, C., 'Qualified Nurses Outwith the Scottish NHS', Institute of Operational Research, Tavistock Institute of Human Relations, London 1977.

Long, A.F. and Cree, J., 'Manpower Information: Case Studies for Training', Health Services Manpower Review, vol.6, no.3, 1980.

Long, A.F. and Mercer, G., 'Nurses Down the Drain: How Bad Planning Wastes Resources', Nursing Mirror, 23 November 1978.

Long, A.F. and Mercer, G., 'NHS Manpower Planning - Towards a Positive Approach?', Health Services Manpower Review, vol.6, nos.2 and 3, 1980.

Long, A.F. and Mercer, G., 'Manpower Planning in the NHS - A Report of a Survey', Nuffield Centre for Health Services Studies, University of Leeds, April 1980.

McCarthy, Lord, Making Whitley Work, DHSS, London 1976.

McLachlan, G. (ed.), Challenges for Change, Nuffield Provincial Hospitals Trust, Oxford University Press, Oxford 1971.

McLachlan, G., Stocking, B. and Shegog, R.F.A. (eds), Patterns for Uncertainty? Planning for the Greater Medical Profession, Nuffield Provincial Hospitals Trust, Oxford University Press, Oxford 1979.

Manson, T., 'Management, the Professions and the Unions', in Stacey, M. et al. (eds), Health and the Division of Labour, Croom Helm, London 1977, pp.196-216.

Maynard, A. and Walker, A., 'A Critical Survey of Medical Manpower Planning in Britain', Social and Economic Administration, vol.11, no.1, 1977, pp.52-75.

Maynard, A. and Walker, A., Doctor Manpower 1975-2000: Alternative Forecasts and Their Resource Implications, Royal Commission on the National Health Service, Research Paper no.4, HMSO, London 1978.

Mejia, A., 'Migration of Physicians and Nurses: A World Wide Picture', International Journal of Epidemiology, vol.7, no.3, 1978, pp.207-215.

Mejia, A., 'The Health Manpower Process', in Hall, T.L. and Mejia, A. (eds), Health Manpower Planning: Principles, Methods, Issues, World Health Organisation, Geneva 1978, pp.31-56.

Mercer, G., The Employment of Nurses, Croom Helm, London 1979.

Mills, A., 'Programme Definition and Programme Budgetting within the NHS Planning System', Nuffield Centre for Health Services Studies, University of Leeds, January 1979.

Ministry of Health and Ministry of Labour and National Service, Staffing the Hospitals - An Urgent National Need, HMSO, London 1945.

Mooney, G., 'Programme Budgetting in an Area Health Board', Hospital and Health Services Review, November 1977, pp.379-384.

National Board for Prices and Incomes, Pay of Nurses and Midwives in the National Health Service, Report no.60, HMSO, London 1968.

National Board for Prices and Incomes, The Pay and Conditions of Manual Workers in Local Authorities, the National Health Service, Gas and Water Supply, Report no.29, HMSO, London 1967.

National Staff Committee for Administrative and Clerical Staff, The Recruitment and Career Development of Administrators, (Hoare Report), DHSS, London 1978.

Nelson, M.J., 'Labour Market Survey', Health Services Manpower Review, vol.2, no.2, 1976.

Nelson, M.J., 'The Market Place for Manpower', Southampton and South West Hampshire Health District, Southampton 1977.

Parry, N. and Parry, J., The Rise of the Medical Profession, Croom Helm, London 1976.

Perrin, J., Management of Financial Resources in the National Health

Service, Royal Commission on the National Health Service, Research
Paper no.2, HMSO, London 1978.

Powell, J.E., A New Look at Medicine and Politics, Pitman, London 1966.

Radical Statistics Health Group, 'A Critique of "Priorities for Health
and Personal Social Services in England"', International Journal of
Health Services, vol.8, no.2, 1978, pp.367-400.

Rafferty, J. (ed.), Health Manpower and Productivity, Heath, Lexington
1974.

Ray, K., 'Manpower Planning - A Systematic Approach', Local Government
Chronicle, 24 June 1977.

Reedy, B.L.E.C., 'Substitution and the Manpower Dilemma', in McLachlan,
G., Stocking, B. and Shegog, R.F.A. (eds), Patterns for Uncertainty?
Planning for the Greater Medical Profession, Nuffield Provincial
Hospitals Trust, Oxford University Press, Oxford 1979, pp.149-164.

Regional Nursing and Midwifery Committee, 'Manpower Planning for Nursing
and Midwifery Staff', South East Thames Regional Health Authority,
March 1979.

Resource Allocation Working Party (RAWP), Sharing Resources for Health
in England, HMSO, London 1976.

Royal Commission on Local Government in England 1966-69, Report, Cmnd.
4040, HMSO, London 1969.

Royal Commission on Medical Education, Report, (Todd Report), Cmnd.
3569, HMSO, London 1978.

Royal Commission on the National Health Service, Report, (Merrison
Report), Cmnd. 7615, HMSO, London 1979.

Royal Commission on the National Health Service, The Task of the
Commission, HMSO, London 1976.

Sadler, J. and Whitworth, T., Resources of Nurses, HMSO, London 1975.

Scott-Samuel, A., 'The Politics of Health', Community Medicine, vol.1,
1979.

Scottish Home and Health Department (SHHD), Nursing Manpower Planning
Reports, nos.1-4, SHHD, Edinburgh 1974-5.

Shegog, R.F.A., 'Manpower Research and the NHS', in McLachlan, G.,
Stocking, B. and Shegog, R.F.A. (eds), Patterns for Uncertainty?
Planning for the Greater Medical Profession, Nuffield Provincial
Hospitals Trust, Oxford University Press, Oxford 1979, pp.185-214.

Shore, E., 'Medical Manpower Planning', Health Trends, vol.6, no.2, May
1974.

Stainer, G., Manpower Planning, Heinemann, London 1971.

Standing Commission on Pay Comparability, (Clegg Commission), Report
No.1 - Local Authority and University Manual Workers, NHS Ancillary
Staffs and Ambulancemen, Cmnd. 7641, HMSO, London 1979.

Stacey, M., Reid, M. and Heath, C. (eds), Health and the Division of
Labour, Croom Helm, London 1977.

Stocking, B., 'Confusion or Control? Manpower in the Complementary
Health Professions', in McLachlan, G., Stocking, B. and Shegog,
R.F.A. (eds), Patterns for Uncertainty? Planning for the Greater
Medical Profession, Nuffield Provincial Hospitals Trust, Oxford
University Press, Oxford 1979, pp.81-136.

The Government's Expenditure Plans 1979-80 to 1982-83, Cmnd. 7439,
HMSO, London 1979.

Trent Regional Health Authority, 'Regional Guidelines for Strategic
Planning 1978-79', Trent Regional Health Authority, April 1978.

Watkin, B., The National Health Service: The First Phase, Allen and
Unwin, London 1978.

Wessex Regional Health Authority, 'Wessex Regional Plan', Paper R529,

Wessex Regional Health Authority, 1979.

West Midlands Regional Health Authority, <u>Regional Strategy 1979-1988</u>, vol.3, West Midlands Regional Health Authority, Birmingham 1979.

Index

References from Notes indicated by 'n' after page reference

staff 9-10, 33-4, 38-42, 93-4, 106, 132-4, 156-7; and planning system 20-1, 85, 102, 104, 116; relations with other tiers 7, 10, 104, 132, 134; see also Joint Manpower Planning and Information Working Group, Manpower Intelligence Branch, National Health Service, Operational Research Service, Standard Manpower Planning and Personnel Information System, and individual staff groups

devolution 12, 96, 111, 114, 121, 132-7, 143-4, 151, 160: and Royal Commission on the National Health Service 11, 97, 133, 152; see also centralisation

direction of staff 84, 133-4, 149-50, 155-7

distribution of manpower 7-8, 34-5, 82, 98n, 108, 133-4, 136

District: future role (and new District Health Authorities) 135, 144, 154-5, 158, 160; manpower planning practice 12, 114, 132, 137-45, 150-2; operational planning, 7, 33-42 passim, 45

Dixon, P. 111, 149

doctors see medical staff

economic: climate in UK 1-2, 10, 148; influences on demand and supply 22, 86; pressures on NHS 2, 8, 10, 13n, 25, 81, 148

education see individual staff groups, and training

engineers 9

Engleman, S.R. 86

European Economic Community (EEC): directives 22, 92, 154

expenditure see National Health Service, and state expenditure

female: participation 87, 154-5, 157; proportion of NHS staff 3, 19, 50

finance see National Health Service

flexibility see staff

focal points 103, 132: future role 113, 158-60; manpower planning practice 111-14; see also Joint Manpower Planning and Information Working Group

forecasting: accuracy 9, 18-19; demand and supply 9, 14-15n, 16-19, 28, 34, 58, 106-9, 112-14; labour turnover 55, 99-100n; see also individual staff groups

Fox, A. 97

geographical mobility 9, 48-9, 89

guidance: Department of Health and Social Security 108-9, 116, 122; Regional Health Authority 113, 117, 136, 154

guidelines see norms

Guillebaud Committee 86

Hall, T.L. 25

Halsbury Committee 82

Harrison, S. 150

health: care and services 1-3, 7, 10, 19, 81, 86-7, 99n, 101, 108, 136, 145, 149, 153, 160-2; inputs and outputs 2, 27; international comparisons 3; see also demand, planning and supply

Hoare Report 10, 107

hospital 38-9, 85: nurse staffing case study 71-4; planning 22, 27; staff numbers 4-5, 86

industrial: disputes 6, 148; relations 18, 86, 89

information 10, 18, 22-4, 45, 63-5, 113, 141-2: base 95, 105-6; problems 28, 44, 64-5, 67, 76-7, 101, 104-5, 113, 141; uses 64, 66, 71-6, 80n; see also manpower information system, Standard Manpower Planning and Personnel Information System

Jay Report 59

Joint Manpower Planning and Information Working Group (MAPLIN): membership 103, 132, 159; role 102-3, 106-9, 112, 152, 158-9; standard classifications 70, 105; see also Standard Manpower Planning and Personnel Information System

Keeling, D. 96

Klein, R. 83

22, 27, 82-3, 98n, 100n, 106;
education and training 90-3,
107, 154; nurse staffing case
study 71-4; see also Briggs
Report, case studies and Salmon
Report

occupational therapists 22, 43-52
passim, 149: see also case
studies
operational: level 7, 10, 107;
research 10, 106; see also
planning
Operational Research Service
(ORS) 106, 108

paramedical staff 4-5, 9, 11,
18-19, 107: central planning
133-5, 144; chiropodists 22,
134; demand and supply 22,
82-3, 90-3, 133; education
and training 90-3, 156;
physiotherapists 100n, 160;
speech therapists 25, 27, 134;
see also case studies, Council
for Professions Supplementary
to Medicine, occupational
therapists and radiographers
part time staff 3, 19, 50, 154,
157
pay 6, 9-10, 89, 155-7, 161
Pay Comparability Commission
6, 89, 105
personnel 10, 68, 101-4:
officers 10, 113, 132, 153,
158, 160-1; role in manpower
planning 113, 138-42, 150, 153,
159-61; see also information
planning 7, 10-11, 19-21, 33, 81,
84, 102-4, 135-6, 143-4;
bottom up 108, 111-12, 116,
121, 134; constraints 24-5,
81, 84, 87, 96, 104; officers
137-142 passim, 150, 153-4;
operational 11, 20-1, 33, 111,
135-6, 143-4, 161; rationality
81, 83, 95-6; strategic 12,
20-1, 28, 40, 59-60, 61n,
102-4, 108, 111-14, 123, 135-6,
138; top down 111-13
Platt Report 82, 86
political pressures in NHS 12,
51, 81-97 passim, 150, 152, 161
pressure groups 85, 88, 91, 97
priorities 8, 10, 20-1, 28, 81,
83, 136, 138, 143-4

private: health care 19, 24;
industry comparison 6-7
productivity 6, 27, 153-5, 157,
160-1: see also work study
professional and technical staff
3-5, 82, 97, 112: see also
paramedical staff
professions 83-7, 92, 94, 101-2,
112, 121, 123, 137, 154-7, 160;
involvement in planning 6, 21,
44, 89, 96, 98n, 137; total
numbers in NHS 3-5, 101-2; see
also individual staff groups

Quirk Report 25, 27

radiographers 82-3, 90-3
ratios see demand measures
recruitment 53-9 passim, 73, 89,
104, 121, 130, 133, 135, 141,
157: difficulties 9, 87-90,
113, 154-5; see also labour
turnover and supply
Regional administrators 1, 14n,
108, 134
Regional Health Authority (RHA) 7,
57, 64, 102-4, 118, 132, 143-4:
demand and supply 41-52 passim,
85, 120-1, 155-7; relations
with other tiers 104-5, 107,
136; strategic planning 111-16,
120-1, 124-5, 128-30; see also
focal points, Resource
Allocation Working Party and
Standard Manpower Planning and
Personnel Information System
reorganisation see National Health
Service
Resource Allocation Working Party
(RAWP) 7, 21, 24-5, 28, 62, 81,
84, 94, 115, 127, 134, 148, 152
restructuring see National Health
Service
Royal Commission on the National
Health Service (Merrison Report)
1-2, 9-12, 19, 27-8, 82, 104-5,
107, 146n: centralisation or
devolution 97, 132-5, 151;
positive approach 2, 12, 113,
133, 145

Salmon Report 7, 10
scientific staff 8, 107
Scottish Home and Health
Department (SHHD) 10, 81, 103
Secretary of State for Social